Histology

Biopsy Pathology
of the Small Intestine

BIOPSY PATHOLOGY SERIES

General Editors:
Professor F. Walker, M.D., Ph.D.
Department of Pathology, University of
Leicester, U.K.

Professor A. Munro Neville, M.D., Ph.D., M.R.C.Path.
Ludwig Institute for Cancer Research,
Sutton, U.K.

Biopsy Pathology
of the Small Intestine

F. D. LEE
M.D., F.R.C.Path.
Consultant Pathologist, Glasgow Royal Infirmary and
Honorary Clinical Lecturer, Glasgow University

AND

P. G. TONER
M.B., Ch.B., D.Sc., M.R.C.Path.
Reader in Pathology, Glasgow University, and Honorary
Consultant Pathologist, Glasgow Royal Infirmary

LONDON
CHAPMAN AND HALL

First published 1980
by Chapman and Hall Ltd
11 New Fetter Lane London EC4P 4EE
© *1980 F. D. Lee and P. G. Toner*
Phototypeset in V.I.P. Palatino by
Western Printing Services Ltd, Bristol
Printed in Great Britain at the
University Press, Cambridge

ISBN 0-412-15060-3

British Library Cataloguing in Publication Data

Lee, F D
 Biopsy pathology of the small intestine. -
 (Biopsy pathology series).
 1. Intestine, Small - Biopsy
 I. Title
 II. Toner, Peter Gilmour
 III. Series
 616.3'4'07583   RC804.B5

 ISBN 0-412-15060-3

Contents

Preface

Since its introduction in 1957, the technique of peroral intestinal biopsy has become a standard investigative procedure in gastroenterology. Nowadays, with increasing frequency, the clinical gastroenterologist looks to the histopathologist for assistance in a growing range of clinical disease, through the interpretation of mucosal biopsies. This book is designed to provide the pathologist with some practical assistance in the interpretation of the histopathology of the intestinal biopsy. The book falls into two broad sections. In the first four chapters, various general topics are discussed such as the physical handling of the biopsy, the use of certain specialized techniques, the structure of the normal mucosa, and the systematic analysis and classification of mucosal abnormalities. The diagnostic and clinical implications of such abnormalities are considered in a general way. In the second part of the book, in Chapters 5–9, there is a detailed description of particular disease processes, with reference to the range of associated pathological changes. This dual approach to the histopathology of the intestinal mucosa involves some repetition of detail. Nevertheless, we believe that this layout is likely to afford the maximum of practical help to the service pathologist, for whom this book is primarily designed.

F. D. Lee
P. G. Toner
Glasgow, January 1979.

Acknowledgements

We are grateful to our many colleagues, both in clinical and laboratory medicine, who have shared with us their thoughts and experience in the field of gastro-intestinal disease. We are indebted to our colleagues in the technical staff for the unfailing support which they have provided at all stages of our work. Particular thanks are due to Mr T. Parker, for the many hours of skilful attention to detail involved in the production of the histological illustrations for this work; to the technical staff of the Electron Microscope Unit for their skilful support in the ultrastructural domain; and to Mrs Riach and her colleagues for endless clerical assistance in the preparation of the manuscript.

Part One:
General considerations

1 Introduction

1.1 The development of biopsy methods

Before the introduction of *in vivo* intestinal biopsy techniques, relatively little was known about the morphology of human intestinal mucosa under normal conditions, and still less about its pathological states. Rapid autolysis renders post-mortem histological examination of the intestinal mucosa difficult and, at times, impossible; and while gross mucosal lesions can be readily studied in surgical resections, the significance of more subtle mucosal changes cannot be readily verified in the absence of unequivocally normal control material. For such reasons, post-mortem histological studies reporting abnormality of the intestinal mucosa in conditions such as tropical sprue (Manson-Bahr, 1924) and adult coeliac disease (Adlersberg and Schein, 1947) were largely disregarded. Similarly, the earlier accounts of 'villous atrophy' in surgical resections of the jejunum in patients with idiopathic steatorrhoea (Paulley, 1954) were not fully appreciated. Even when the first biopsy studies confirmed these findings, it took some time before their importance was accepted unreservedly.

The first intestinal biopsies were carried out with a modification of the rigid gastric biopsy tube, (Shiner, 1956) and it was only after the introduction of the much more flexible biopsy capsule (Crosby and Kugler, 1957) that the technique of intestinal biopsy became extensively used throughout the world (Greene *et al.*, 1974; Townley and Barnes, 1973). Further developments have enhanced the value of the procedure by making it possible to take multiple biopsies from different parts of the intestinal tract. The numerous studies of the intestinal mucosa that have resulted are reviewed in various papers and books (Rubin and Dobbins, 1965; Whitehead, 1973; Creamer, 1974; Perera *et al.*, 1975). The recently introduced modern techniques of endoscopy have added yet another dimension to the investigation of intestinal disease: biopsy of the proximal duodenum is now generally carried out under direct visualization and even the terminal ileum has become accessible to biopsy with the colonoscope. The biopsy capsule, however, remains the most convenient instrument for sampling the greater part of the small intestine. It can, moreover, be used not only for the histological and ultrastructural assessment of the intestinal mucosa but also for the analysis of intestinal enzymes and for the sampling of the bacterial flora which inhabit the intestinal lumen.

1.2 The limitations of biopsy

It has been recognized that intestinal biopsy has important limitations. In the first place only the mucosa and, at most, the superficial part of the submucosa are included in the material sampled. This means that only disease which primarily or predominantly affects the mucosa is likely to be detected. Conditions such as Crohn's disease, in which the distinctive lesions are usually found more deeply in the bowel wall, cannot as a rule be confidently diagnosed. Secondly, biopsy is only likely to be of value in those disease states in which the lesions are sufficiently diffuse to be sampled on a random basis. The only exceptions to this are diseases of the proximal duodenum or terminal ileum, in which the lesions can be directly visualized by endoscopic techniques. It has also to be appreciated that even in 'diffuse' diseases the lesions may vary in severity. Mucosal change is always most marked at the exposed extremities of the mucosal folds, and may be minimal or even absent in the 'troughs' between the folds. The possibility of sampling error must always be considered when a biopsy is found to be normal against clinical expectation: in such instances repeat biopsy is advisable before treatment, which may be lifelong, is instituted. A third problem common to all biopsy procedures, but especially troublesome in intestinal biopsies, is the difficulty of defining the limits of normality in morphological terms. The intestinal mucosa shows a remarkably wide range of variation under apparently normal conditions: there can be no doubt that in many instances the minor pathological changes described in a variety of diseases have been spurious, while on the other hand it is possible that minor changes of potential significance have been ignored. While experience is helpful in this respect, there is obviously a need to develop more discriminating methods of assessing biopsies.

1.3 The indications for biopsy

Malabsorption is by far the most important indication for intestinal biopsy and the greater part of this book is devoted to the histopathology of the intestinal mucosal manifestations of malabsorptive conditions. In Western communities, where coeliac disease is one of the most common causes of malabsorption at almost any age, the value of biopsy is now unquestioned; indeed it is regarded by many as the single most important diagnostic test in the investigation of malabsorptive disorders. In tropical or underdeveloped countries, where coeliac disease is much less important than certain other causes of malabsorption such as pancreatic insufficiency, the value of biopsy is less well established. Moreover, the particularly wide variation in normal morphology observed in the tropics creates special problems in biopsy interpretation, and pathological changes must be reported with more than the usual degree of caution.

Apart from primary malabsorptive disturbances, intestinal biopsy is only rarely of help in the diagnosis of other intestinal diseases. With the exception of the diffuse lymphomas of so-called Mediterranean type and tumours of the proximal duodenum, which can be directly visualized by endoscopy, an intestinal neoplasm would only be sampled by biopsy and confidently diagnosed by chance. The same is true of most cases of Crohn's disease. Infectious disease and helminthic infestation may both, it is true, be detected by biopsy techniques. Interesting results have been obtained in this way in the investigation of acute gastroenteritis of childhood, but in general non-invasive methods of diagnosis are to be preferred in such cases. Intestinal biopsy may be useful in the diagnosis of certain multi-system diseases even if symptoms referable to the intestinal tract are not evident. The most obvious example of this is amyloid disease. In some such diseases however, the more readily accessible colonic mucosa is also affected and is a more convenient biopsy site.

1.4 The scope of the book

In this book the pathology of intestinal biopsies has been approached in two different ways. First, the types of pathological response of which the intestine, and in particular the intestinal mucosa is capable are described and defined insofar as this is possible, and the diagnostic implications of these responses are briefly considered. Secondly, the pathological features of the principal disease processes which affect the small bowel are systematically described in greater detail. Emphasis is placed on those conditions which are most likely to be detected by intestinal biopsy, although diseases which may be encountered by chance in biopsy material have also been included. This dual approach has been adopted because it is thought to correspond to the two main practical problems most often faced by a pathologist in the laboratory: is a particular histological alteration pathologically significant, and what are the diagnostic possibilities?; and what are the pathological changes which may be associated with a particular clinically suspected disease process? If the text is to respond to both of these questions, some degree of repetition is inevitable and may even on occasion be desirable: nevertheless it has been kept to a minimum wherever possible.

Finally, while most of the information in this book relates to histopathology, the importance of other methods of biopsy assessment is recognized and various conditions are identified in which specialized techniques such as electron microscopy have proved of interest or are likely to yield additional information. We hope that the book will serve not only as a practical aid to the diagnostic pathologist, but also as a stimulus to the further study of the intestinal biopsy in the context of clinical research.

References

Adlersberg, D. and Schein, J. (1947), Clinical and pathological studies in sprue. *J. Am. med. Ass.*, 134, 1459–1467.

Creamer, B. (1974), *The small intestine*. Heinemann Medical Books, London.

Crosby, W. H. and Kugler, H. W. (1957), Intraluminal biopsy of the small intestine: the intestinal biopsy capsule. *Am. J. dig. Dis.*, 2, 236–241.

Greene, H. L., Rosensweig, N. S., Lufkin, E. G., Hagler, L., Gozansky, D., Taunton, O. D. and Herman, R. H. (1974), Biopsy of the small intestine with the Crosby-Kugler capsule. Experience in 3866 peroral biopsies in children and adults. *Am. J. dig. Dis.*, 19, 189–198.

Manson-Bahr, P. (1924), Morbid anatomy and pathology of sprue, and their bearing upon aetiology. *Lancet*, 1, 1148–1151.

Paulley, J. W. (1954), Observations on the aetiology of idiopathic steatorrhoea. Jejunal and lymph node biopsies. *Br. med. J.*, 2, 1318–1321.

Perera, D., Weinstein, W. M. and Rubin, C. E. (1975), Small intestinal biopsy. *Human Pathol.*, 6, 157–217.

Rubin, C. E. and Dobbins, W. O. (1965), Peroral biopsy of the small intestine. A review of its diagnostic usefulness. *Gastroenterology*, 49, 676–697.

Shiner, M. (1956), Jejunal biopsy tube. *Lancet*, 1, 85.

Townley, R. R. W. and Barnes, G. L. (1973), Intestinal biopsy in childhood. *Archs. Dis. Childh.*, 48, 480–482.

Whitehead, R. (1973), *Mucosal biopsy of the gastrointestinal tract*. W. B. Saunders, London.

2 The handling of biopsies

2.1 The biopsy capsule

Apart from the most proximal part of the duodenum and the most distal part of the ileum, which have recently become accessible to biopsy under direct visualization by endoscopic techniques, biopsy of the small intestine is carried out on a random basis. A suction capsule such as the instrument developed by Crosby and Kugler in 1957 is still widely used; and although many modifications, including the facility for multiple biopsy, have since been introduced, the basic mechanism remains unchanged. After the instrument has been introduced and its position in the upper jejunum verified radiologically, suction is applied to draw the intestinal mucosa through an orifice in the capsule: subsequent release of a spring-loaded knife cuts off the aspirated knuckle of mucosa, which is then trapped within the capsule. If the procedure is carried out correctly it is safe and reliable, and trauma both to the patient and to the biopsy is minimal. It is important, however, that the biopsy should be recovered as soon as possible. Autolysis of the intestinal mucosa is extremely rapid, and more than a few minutes' delay may seriously prejudice the diagnostic value of the procedure.

While biopsies of the intestinal mucosa can be assessed by a number of different methods, the only one which is indispensable is histological examination. If for no other reason than to identify the source of a biopsy, the greatest attention must always be given to this. Other methods may, however, be of value when certain intestinal disease processes are suspected; for this reason it is important that the diagnostic possibilities should be considered by the clinician before a biopsy is taken so that the appropriate facilities are available at the right time. The discussion of laboratory methods which follows is thus not without relevance to clinicians.

2.2 Dissecting microscopy

This is routinely used in Britain as a means of obtaining a 'three-dimensional' assessment of mucosal architecture. Its value is, however, limited and a diagnosis should never be made until histological confirmation is available. The procedure has to be carried out as soon as possible after the biopsy has been extruded from the capsule, to avoid delay before the material is placed in fixative. For optimal dissecting microscope assessment (and subsequent fixation) the biopsy should be carefully layered on to a small portion of cardboard or blotting-paper with the submucosal surface, of course, facing downwards. This is not always as easy as it sounds, since the villous surface in some diseases is flat and apparently structureless, or the villi may be obscured by mucus. If there is any doubt, it is better not to attach the biopsy to paper and to place it instead directly into fixative, accepting the consequences of this – such as curling and distortion – as the lesser of two evils. Any manipulation of the villous surface, even that involved in teasing out mucus, is to be deprecated. The only exception to this rule is in suspected cases of giardiasis, since the organisms are most readily detected in smears of mucus stained by the Giemsa method. The 'layered' biopsy is immersed in normal saline for examination under the dissecting microscope for which incident light is usually preferable. Fixed biopsies can also be examined under the dissecting microscope although the distortion and shrinkage caused by the fixative is liable to exaggerate any abnormality that may be present.

The results of dissecting microscopy, expressed in simple descriptive terms, are of course purely subjective unless biopsies are routinely photographed. Many observers find grading systems useful in recording results, especially in research studies, and one such system is illustrated in Table 2.1. It has to be noted, however, that only grade V –

Table 2.1 Dissecting microscope appearances of the jejunal mucosa (modified from Stanfield *et al.*, 1965).

Grade	Appearance
I	Finger villi only
II	Leaf villi only, or leaf and finger villi
III	Leaf villi with some fusion to form small ridges or convolutions
IV	Convolutions or ridging with no recognizable villi – often some flattening
V	Notable flattening of the mucosa with no recognizable pattern topographically

the completely 'flat' jejunal biopsy – is unequivocally abnormal in all parts of the world. Grades I to III can all be seen in apparently normal individuals, and in tropical countries even grade IV is not necessarily pathological (Section 3.2).

2.3 Histological processing and examination

It has often been emphasized, and with good reason, that the processing of biopsies for histology is a matter of considerable importance. As mentioned previously, the attachment of biopsies to paper or cardboard before fixation prevents distortion and is generally recommended whether dissecting microscopy is carried out or not. With small biopsies – such as those obtained by endoscopic techniques – the value of this is debatable since the advantages may be outweighed by the trauma produced by manipulation of the biopsy during attachment.

The fixative employed is largely a matter of personal preference. Many pathologists favour Bouin's fluid (picric acid – acetic acid – formalin) which facilitates section cutting and produces less tissue shrinkage than formol-saline. Bouin's fluid does, however, have some disadvantages. It tends for example to destroy some cytoplasmic granules, especially those which characterize Paneth cells. Formol-saline is probably still the most widely used general fixative in this country and for this reason most of the illustrations have been prepared from formalin-fixed material. Whether or not it is better to process all the fixed material for histology, or to retain a part of the biopsy in fixative should the need for fat stains or belated electron microscopy arise, is again a matter of judgement. In the great majority of cases, however, assessment of mucosal architecture is the primary objective and the need for a well-orientated biopsy is paramount. The subdivision of a biopsy into fragments is best avoided if it adds difficulty to the orientation of the material prior to the embedding procedure, which is a critically important step in biopsy processing. The pathologist should orientate the material personally at this stage; he cannot then blame the technical staff if things go wrong. Even with accurately embedded material, a biopsy then has to be cut at several levels before a section is obtained which is satisfactorily orientated at right angles to the lamina muscularis mucosae. This is most readily assessed from the appearance of the crypts of Lieberkuhn, which should be visible throughout their entire length (Fig. 3.4).

2.4 Staining procedures

In the great majority of cases, a standard haemalum-eosin (HE) is all that is required for diagnostic purposes. Further staining procedures are, however, sometimes useful and occasionally essential, as will become evident when specific disease processes are discussed. Only a brief summary regarding the value of special stains will be given here.

The periodic acid-Schiff (P.A.S.) method beautifully demonstrates the brush border of enterocytes, the mucus of goblet cells and lipofuscin pigmentation of smooth muscle (Section 4.1.3). Its particular value lies in the detection of the abnormal histiocytic infiltration which characterizes Whipple's disease (Section 6.1), rare cases of fungal infection of the intestinal tract and the confirmation of gastric metaplasia in the villous epithelium of the proximal duodenum (Section 4.12). Masson's trichrome technique is occasionally helpful in demonstrating muscle fibres, collagen formation or fibrin deposition in the intestinal mucosa, and stains Paneth cells brilliantly. Like the P.A.S., however, it is not necessary as a routine procedure; furthermore, Lendrum's Martius Scarlet-blue (M.S.B.; Lendrum *et al.*, 1962) is preferable for the recognition of fibrin, and Lendrum's phloxine – tartrazine (Lendrum, 1947) gives an even more impressive demonstration of Paneth cells, as well as being useful in the detection of viral inclusion bodies. Reticulin stains, of which the phospho-tannin silver impregnation method (Slidders, Fraser and Lendrum, 1958) has been found most satisfactory, are sometimes required, especially in the assessment of lymphoproliferative states. The methyl green pyronin (MGP) stain for ribonucleic acid is also useful in assessing intestinal lymphomas, many of which show plasma cell differentiation. This stain may also be useful in detecting the presence or absence of plasma cells in the lamina propria, especially in cases of suspected immunodeficiency (Section 5.5). The argentaffin, diazo and argyrophil reactions are mandatory in suspected tumours of the APUD system (carcinoid tumours). Mucin stains, such as Alcian blue or P.A.S. are sometimes useful in the diagnosis of epithelial tumours. Sections stained wth Thioflavine -T or Sirius red, and examined under UV-light or polarized light respectively, are essential to confirm the presence of amyloid, and should perhaps be used more often than is at present the case. The polarizing microscope should also be used as a routine in the examination sarcoid – like granulomatous lesions, and it need hardly be added that a Ziehl-Neelsen (Z.N.) stain for acid- and alcohol-fast bacilli is mandatory in such cases. Non-iron-containing pigments belonging to the general category of lipofuscin can usually be identified in H.E. sections, by virtue of their position in muscle cells (Fig. 4.35); for confirmation, the 'long acid-fast' modification of ZN, or, as mentioned above, the P.A.S. stain, are helpful. When any form of pathological pigmentation in the intestine is suspected it is essential to test for haemosiderin by employing the classical Perl's Prussian blue reaction with adequate control sections to exclude artefact. With the exception of the rare malabsorptive disease abetalipoproteinaemia (Section 6.3), stains for neutral lipid such as Sudan III and IV or Sudan black B applied to frozen sections are seldom indicated.

While assessment of the immunological status of the intestinal tract is becoming increasingly important (Ferguson and McSween, 1976), a detailed account of the techniques used for this purpose is beyond the scope of this book. In any case most of these techniques are only available in specialized centres. An exception is the immunoperoxidase method (Taylor, 1974) which has an important advantage over other immunohistochemical techniques in that it can be applied to formalin-fixed, paraffin-embedded tissue. This method is becoming increasingly used in the identification of cell products in histological sections (Burns, 1978). Its main application in gastro-intestinal pathology is in the demonstration of immunoglobulin-containing cells (see Isaacson and Wright, 1978); variations in the number and distribution of plasma cells producing different classes of immunoglobulin in the lamina propria are readily detected. By using antisera specific for the kappa or lambda light chains of immunoglobulin it is possible to determine whether a plasma cell infiltrate is polyclonal and thus reactive (both light chains detected) or monoclonal and presumably neoplastic (only one light chain detected). Other uses of the technique include the identification of specific hormone products in tumours of the intestinal endocrine system (Section 9.4).

2.5 Morphometric methods of histological assessment

While subjective visual assessment of a well-prepared histological section is all that is required for routine diagnostic purposes, most pathologists hold the view that histological measurement of one kind or another might be of value in certain circumstances. Morphometric methods have, for example, been shown to be of use in the detection of minor histological abnormalities and may have an important part to play in the classification of villous abnormality or in determining its pathogenesis; they are also essential in research studies which involve direct comparison between experimental groups. The main criticisms levelled at morphometric methods are that they are time-consuming, difficult to standardize and inaccurate due to uncontrollable variations in the fixation or processing of biopsies; some also require specialized equipment which is not generally available. For these reasons, discussion will be limited to those methods which are relatively simple and easily applied in any routine diagnostic laboratory, although it is appreciated that more refined and accurate methods may be required for research purposes.

Most morphometric techniques have been developed for the assessment of villous architecture and in particular for the detection of 'villous atrophy' or reduced absorptive surface area. This latter variable cannot of course be measured directly in biopsies unless elaborate stereological techniques are employed: and even then measurements from a random biopsy sample can never provide more than the vaguest estimate of the functional absorptive area of the small bowel. The modified linear intercept technique of Dunnill and Whitehead (1972), an indirect method for estimating absorptive surface, is reported to be rapid and useful. The critical measurement obtained is the ratio of mucosal surface to volume; visually unimpressive degrees of 'villous atrophy' can be convincingly demonstrated. This ratio does not indicate the pathogenesis of the villous alteration, although this may be deduced from variations in mucosal volume, which can also be measured by this method.

Another method which has been used by many workers (e.g. Shiner and Doniach, 1960) in both clinical and experimental studies is simple measurement of villous height and crypt height using a calibrated micrometer eyepiece. While this has been criticized on the grounds that fixation and processing may influence the results in an unpredictable fashion or that the 'end-points' of measurement are difficult to define due to villous folding or other factors, it has proved to be useful over many years of personal experience. It is of course essential that the biopsy is well-orientated, and at least 10 villi must be measured for valid results. The villous height (VH) is taken as the distance between villous extremity and villous base, judged to be that point on the epithelial surface at which the villous epithelium curves on to the horizontal plane. (Fig. 3.4). When two such points are visible, the mean of the two possible measurements is taken. The crypt height (CH) is taken as the distance between the crypt base and the horizontal epithelial surface at the villous base. In completely 'flat' biopsies, villi appear to be absent and the only clear measurement possible is the total mucosal height (TH) from crypt base to flat epithelial surface (Fig. 4.39); some estimate of VH and CH in such 'flat' biopsies is possible, however, if it is assumed that the dividing point between villous and crypt epithelium is marked by the upper limit of mitotic activity in the mucosa. Calculation of the CH: VH ratio is critically important: this value broadly corresponds to the surface to volume ratio and is unaffected by fixation artefact. The use of these measurements in the classification of villous abnormality is described in Section 4.2.

Morphometric methods may also be used to measure other variable histological features. Eyepiece graticules have been used to estimate the density of leucocytic infiltration and the distribution of leucocytic types within the lamina propria (Holmes *et al.*, 1973), a technique of potential value in detecting premalignant mucosal change (see Section 5.1). Simple measurement of the ratio between intra-epithelial lymphocytes and epithelial cells in ultrathin histological sections (Ferguson and Murray, 1971) may have interesting applications, especially in assessing the activity of coeliac disease (Section 5.1). Measurement of epithelial-cell (enterocyte) height by micrometer eyepiece may also be useful in the investigation of some aspects of coeliac disease. These methods, however, while valuable in research, are probably too time-consuming to be routinely used in the diagnostic assessment of intestinal biopsies.

2.6 Electron microscopy

Ultrastructural examination cannot be said to play an important part in the routine diagnosis of intestinal disease, but its contribution to the understanding of intestinal function and malfunction has been substantial. There is now, however, a growing interest in the fine structural aspects of disease with an increasing involvement of the electron microscopist in biopsy studies. For this reason a brief summary of the technical demands and limitations of electron microscopy is presented, since the responsibility for the organization, if not the performance, of electron microscopy often falls upon the nearest pathologist in such situations.

2.6.1 Procedures for conventional transmission electron microscopy

Often only a single biopsy specimen will be available, necessitating the division of the sample for different laboratory investigations. The requirements of conventional tissue diagnosis must always be met first, if necessary at the expense of the more research-orientated ultrastructural investigation. In most cases, however, a thin strip can generally be cut from the edge of a biopsy without greater tissue loss than is usually incurred in the process of facing the block for histopathological sectioning. The ideal block for electron microscopy is less than 1 mm across, amounting to only a small group of villi. A thin strip of tissue is equally acceptable, provided that the maximum thickness is less than 1 mm. A strip of mucosa has an added advantage over small random blocks, in that the tissue surface can be accurately orientated by the use of an oblong embedding mould, allowing sections to be cut through the long axes of villi and adjacent crypts. The ultrastructural features of the intestine vary so much from crypt base to villous tip that it is essential to know the exact location of an ultrathin section if its interpretation is to be valid.

The handling and trimming of the biopsy must be carried out with the greatest of care, since crush artefacts are particularly damaging to fine structure. Fresh new razor blades must be used, the specimen being placed for trimming on dental wax, which will not dull the cutting edge. Speed is essential, since modifications of fine structure become increasingly evident after the severing of the tissue from its blood supply. With intestinal biopsies one must always keep in mind the additional concealed period of ischaemia from the time the capsule is fired to its withdrawal. There is no 'acceptable' period of fixation delay for electron microscopy – any delay will have some effect, although usually of a minor degree if the delay is limited to a minute or two.

The fixative most widely used today is glutaraldehyde, at concentrations from 1 per cent to 4 per cent in buffer solution at physiological pH. Details of suitable fixative and buffer combinations can be obtained from standard reference works on ultrastructural technique. Stock diluted fixative should be stored at 4°C, and renewed regularly. Ideally the pH should be checked and adjusted if necessary before use. When biopsies are only infrequently taken for electron microscopy, it is better to have fresh fixative made up from concentrated stock solutions just prior to use. Glutaraldehyde fixation interferes with the normal histological tissue processing and staining reactions, so that it is best to separate the main biopsy sample before placing the electron microscopy sample in fixative, although glutaradehyde – formaldehyde mixtures have been proposed which are compatible for both conventional and ultrastructural purposes. (Trump and Jones, 1978.) If individual attention cannot be given to each biopsy, fixatives such as this should be considered, allowing electron microscopy sampling to be carried out at leisure. The edges of a biopsy will generally show the best preservation of tissue ultrastructure in these circumstances. Tissues may remain in fixative for any convenient time, although 2 hours is generally allowed. If long-term storage is required, buffer solution at 4°C should be used.

Tissue processing for electron microscopy is probably best handled in the laboratory responsible for the examination of the tissues, although the procedures are simple and in principle can be followed by any laboratory. In summary, the tissue is post-fixed in 1 per cent osmium tetroxide solution, dehydrated in ethanol, cleared in propylene oxide, and embedded in a suitable resin material such as araldite, epon or spurr medium. Wide variations in cutting properties can be introduced by minor changes in procedure, and liason is necessary between the processing laboratory and the section-cutting laboratory to ensure satisfactory results. Semithin (1 μm) toluidine blue-stained sections are taken for orientation, and ultrathin sections (0.05 μm) are then cut from suitable areas. Contrast enhancement for electron microscopy involves the use of solutions of uranyl and lead salts. The importance of positive identification of the exact location of the area examined cannot be over-emphasized, particularly in studies involving point-counting or other mensuration, which are now becoming more widely used in electron microscopy.

2.6.2 Special ultrastructural techniques

These procedures outlined above are the routine techniques used for thin section work. For special research purposes, other techniques may be appropriate, such as tissue micro-analysis and scanning electron microscopy.

Tissue micro-analysis is achieved by examining the spectrum of X rays produced from the specimen by the electron beam in the electron microscope. The spectrum is displayed as a histogram, plotting the varying numbers of X rays of different energies, varying usually from 0–40 keV. Each element has a characteristic spectrum, or set of peaks, which allow its presence to be recorded, the height of the peaks being roughly proportional to the concentration of the element in the tissue. The techniques for X-ray analysis are still in the development stages, but useful results can now be obtained routinely if adequate concentrations of the elements of interest are present in the tissue. Many complications must be kept in mind, such as artefacts of fixation, the diffusion of certain elements and the leaching out of many substances during processing. In many instances, ultrathin frozen sections may be required to provide a more realistic and meaningful sample for analysis.

Scanning electron microscopy has recently become popular on account of the unique image clarity which is characteristic of this technique (Hodges and Hallowes, 1979). The deeply contoured gut mucosa is particularly amenable to scanning electron microscopy, allowing the full use of its high resolution potential and of its great depth of field (Toner and Carr, 1969; Marsh, 1972). The scanning microscope is at its best in the examination of natural surfaces: it can take specimens of the full thickness of the intestinal mucosa, and up to 10 mm or more in diameter. Thin sections are not necessary for such studies of the mucosal surface. The microscope can record images at any magnification from 20x to 100 000x, with resolution around 5 nm in suitable circumstances and with modern instruments. Recent developments promise scanning resolution equivalent to the level of high resolution transmission electron microscopy, by the use of modern advanced technology equipment.

The scanning electron microscope is quite different in principle from the conventional transmission electron microscope. The electron beam is focussed to a fine point on the specimen surface, and is then deflected to and fro by scanning coils, tracing out, line by line, a square grid pattern or raster on the specimen surface. Secondary electron emission from the surface is picked up by detectors, amplified and displayed on a cathode ray tube, line by line, synchronously with the scanning of the specimen surface. There are no image-forming lenses and the image points are formed successively in time, being integrated into a topographical view of the specimen surface through TV electronics. The resolution is limited by the size of the scanning spot and the ratio of the meaningful signal to the background noise in the system.

For practical purposes, the fixation requirements for scanning electron microscopy can be regarded as identical to those for transmission electron microscopy. Since scanning electron microscopy is ideally suited for the study of large specimens, there is no need to trim the tissue, except to ensure an adequate sample for histopathology. The subsequent handling of the biopsy is best carried out in a specialist laboratory. Osmium impregnation is usually employed followed by either freeze-drying or critical-point drying, both of which avoid the damaging effects of transient air-liquid interfaces during drying. The surface tension forces generated by such adverse drying effects cause serious distortion of fine surface detail. The dried specimen is glued to a specimen carrier with a conducting adhesive such as silver paint, and is then vacuum-coated with a conducting metallic layer to ensure conductivity. These precautions limit the build-up of static change on the specimen surface, which can cause image distortion. Fuller details of this technique and its application can be found in specialist texts, such as the proceedings of the annual Scanning Electron Microscopy symposia held in the U.S.A.

References

Burns, J. (1978), Immunological methods and their applications in the routine laboratory. In *Recent advances in Histopathology*. (Ed. Anthony, P. P. and Woolf, N.), 10th Edition. Churchill Livingstone, Edinburgh.

Crosby, W. H. and Kugler, H. W. (1957), Intraluminal biopsy of the small intestine: the intestinal biopsy capsule. *Am. J. dig. Dis.*, 2, 236–241.

Dunnill, M. S. and Whitehead, R. (1972), A method for the quantitation of small intestinal biopsy specimens. *J. clin. Path.*, 243–246.

Ferguson, A., and McSween, R.N.M. (1976), *Immunological aspects of the liver and gastrointestinal tract*. M.T.P. Press, Lancaster, England.

Ferguson, A. and Murray, D. (1971), Quantitation of intraepithelial lymphocytes in human jejunum. *Gut*, 12, 988–994.

Hodges, G. M. and Hallowes, R. C. (Eds) (1979), *Biomedical applications of scanning electron microscopy*. Academic Press, London.

Holmes, G. K. T., Asquith, P., Stokes, P. J. and Cooke, W. T. (1973), Cellular infiltrate of jejunal biopsies in adult coeliac disease in relation to gluten withdrawal. *Gut*, 14, 429. (Abstract)

Isaacson, P. and Wright, D. H. (1978), Intestinal lymphoma associated with malabsorption. *Lancet*, 1, 67–70.

Lendrum, A. C. (1947), The phloxin-tartrazine method as a general histological stain and for the demonstration of inclusion bodies. *J. Path. Bact.*, 59, 399–404.

Lendrum, A. C., Fraser, D. S., Slidders, W. and Henderson, R. (1962), Studies on the character and staining of fibrin. *J. clin. Path.*, 15, 401–413.

Marsh, M. N. (1972), The scanning electron microscope and its application to the investigation of intestinal structure. In *Recent Advances in Gastroenterology*, (Ed. Badenoch, J. and Brook, B. N.) pp. 81–135. Churchill Livingstone, Edinburgh.

Shiner, M. and Doniach, I. (1960), Histopathologic studies in steatorrhoea. *Gastroenterology*, 38, 419–440.

Slidders, W., Fraser, D. S. and Lendrum, A. C. (1958), Silver impregnation of reticulin. *J. Path. Bact.*, 75, 478–481.

Stanfield, J. P., Hutt, M.S.R. and Tunnicliffe, R. (1965), Intestinal biopsy in kwashiorkor. *Lancet*, 2, 519–523.

Taylor, C. R. (1974), The nature of Reed-Sternberg cells and other malignant 'reticulum' cells. *Lancet*, 2, 802–807.

Toner, P. G. and Carr, K. E. (1966), The use of scanning electron microscopy in the study of the intestinal villi. *J. Pathol.*, 97, 611–617.

Trump, B. F. and Jones, R. T. (1978), *Diagnostic electron microscopy*. John Wiley and Sons, New York.

3 The normal intestinal mucosa

3.1 The mucosal compartments

The unique histological structure of the mucosa of the small intestine is due to the presence of two main compartments. First, there is the functional absorptive compartment normally consisting of tall regular finger-like villi, covered for the most part by absorptive epithelial cells or 'enterocytes'. Secondly, there is a basal compartment occupied largely by the crypts of Lieberkuhn. These are simple tubular gland-like structures, the luminal orifices of which are grouped around the bases of villi. Most of the cells lining the crypts are maturing or dividing enterocyte precursor cells or 'enteroblasts'. The three-dimensional architecture of the intestinal mucosa is most readily appreciated by the use of the dissecting microscope (Section 2.2) or the scanning electron microscope (Fig. 3.1).

With the scanning electron microscope, the fine detail of the villous surface is easily resolved, while the remarkable depth of focus of the instrument allows the re-entrant contours of the mucosa to be fully appreciated. Shallow surface grooves cross the villus, forming an irregular mosaic pattern: similar contours are found on other mucosal surfaces (Fig. 3.2). At higher magnification a polygonal patchwork pattern can be made out. This corresponds to the surface territories of individual enterocytes, the occasional interspersed goblet cell appearing as a pock-mark or indentation, breaking the otherwise relatively smooth contours. At higher magnification still, the individual micro-

---

Fig. 3.1 Human jejunal biopsy showing the comparison between dissecting microscopy (a) and scanning microscopy (b). The dissecting micrograph is characterized by its relatively low resolution of detail and by the relative lack of depth of field. The scanning micrograph on the other hand shows high resolution detail as well as a very striking depth of field. Scanning micrograph by courtesy of Dr K. E. Carr.

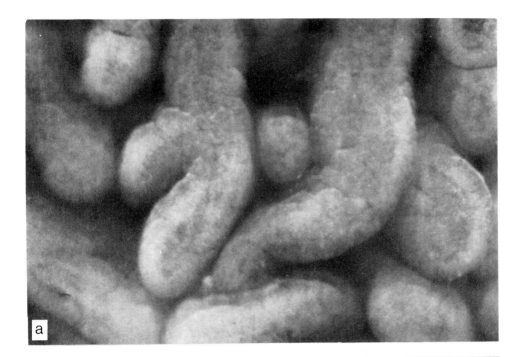

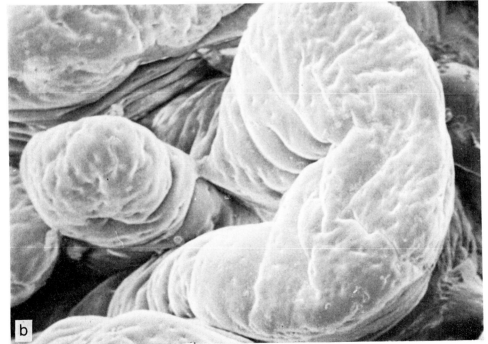

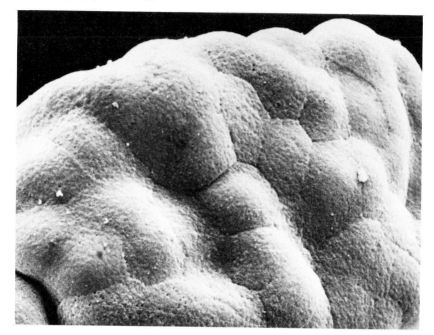

Fig. 3.2 Scanning micrograph of surface of intestinal villus. The polygonal patchwork pattern clearly seen here represents the surface outlines of individual columnar enterocytes. Scanning micrograph by courtesy of Dr K. E. Carr.

villi may be distinguished (Anderson and Taylor, 1973). This is more easily achieved in some species than in others, perhaps because of the variations in the surface fuzzy coat of the enterocytes, which forms a blanket over the tips of the microvilli.

Forming the villous core and surrounding the crypts is the lamina propria mucosae, which consists mainly of supportive connective tissue elements enclosing blood vessels, lymphatics, lymphoreticular cells and a variety of other leucocytes: the lamina propria is separated from the submucosa by a thin double-layered structure known as the lamina muscularis mucosae. This last structure, together with the superficial part of the submucosa, is usually included in jejunal biopsies and may help to sustain the normal mucosal architecture. Certainly, it is worth noting that when the lamina is not present, the villi may become unduly separated and stunted in appearance giving a false impression of abnormality.

The extent to which mucosal morphology varies in apparently normal individuals within a given community cannot be over-emphasized and must always be taken into account in biopsy interpretation. There is, moreover, a substantial geographical variation in mucosal morphology. The cause of this is unkown, although it appears to be related more to climatic and perhaps dietary considerations (Owen and Brandborg, 1977) than to ethnic factors. Mucosal morphology has been observed to change when a normal individual moves from a temperate to a tropical environment (Lindenbaum *et al.*, 1966). This phenomenon is not without diagnostic importance, since the mucosal appearances found in some normal individuals resident in the tropics would be regarded as distinctly abnormal in a temperate climate (Mathan *et al.*, 1975). These individual and geographical variations must therefore be included in any discussion of normal morphology and if possible should be incorporated into the histological definition of normality (see Section 3.6).

3.2 Mucosal architecture

In temperate climates, the jejunal villi are for the most part tall, slender and finger-shaped when viewed under the dissecting microscope. Usually, however, a small proportion of the villi are broader and leaf-shaped (Fig. 3.3) and even short ridges are found on occasion in apparently normal biopsies. Such atypical villous forms are more often found in the proximal parts of the duodenum (Booth *et al.*, 1962). On the other hand, in the ileum, the villi tend to be even taller and more slender than in the jejunum (Steward *et al.*, 1967). Histologically, the villi are regularly disposed and measure on average between 300 μm and 500 μm in height; a villous height of less than 300 μm should be regarded as abnormal. The villi vary little in width from base to apex, and the mean width is usually less than 150 μm (Fig. 3.4). The broader, irregularly-shaped or branched villi occasionally seen probably represent leaf villi sectioned in various planes. The crypts of Lieberkuhn are of simple tubular structure and are regular in distribution: they vary in height from 110 μm to 230 μm (mean 170 μm) and it is of importance to note that the ratio of crypt height to villous height does not exceed 0.6 under normal conditions; on average this ratio is about two-fifths (0.4).

In the tropics, a substantially different picture has emerged. Under the dissecting microscope finger villi are much less conspicuous than in 'temperate' biopsies; the leaf villus is the predominant form and is quite often accompanied by short ridges and even on occasion a convoluted pattern. Histologically, the villi tend to have a pyramidal shape, being broader at the base than at the apex (Fig. 3.5). They are also significantly shorter than their temperate counterparts and measure anything between 150 μm and 430 μm in height. In terms of villous

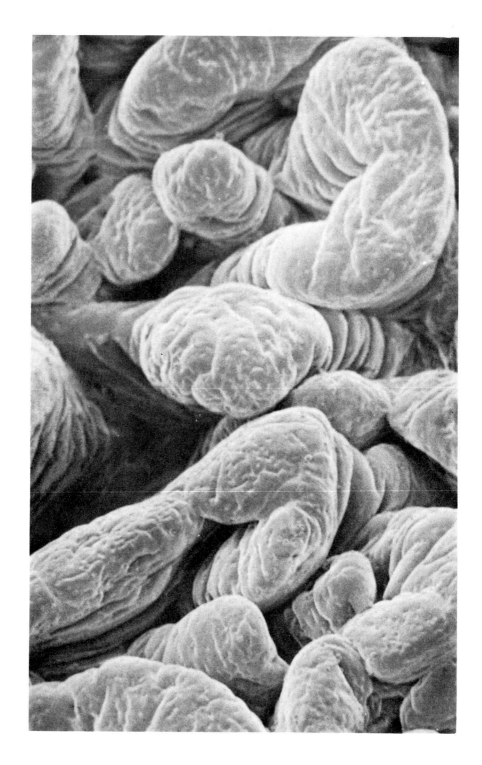

height, at least half of all tropical biopsies would be regarded as abnormal by temperate standards. On the other hand the villous width tends to be greater, and mean measurements of over 200 μm are by no (mean 0.45) and is thus similar to that of the temperate normal. The high proportion of leaf villi. The crypt height, however, is reduced in proportion to villous height (range 100–195 μm; mean 130 μm) with the result that the ratio of crypt height to villous height rarely exceeds 0.6 (mean 0.45) and is thus similar to that of the temperate normal. The results of measurements personally carried out in temperate and tropical biopsies are summarized in Table 3.1.

Table 3.1 Mucosal measurements (mean, standard deviation, and range) in normal jejunal biopsies (Lee, 1970).

Variable	'Temperate' normal (Britain: 24 cases)		'Tropical' normal (East Africa: 35 cases)	
Villous height μm	413	± 52 (313–512)	311	± 63 (155–431)
Crypt height μm	169	± 29 (114–231)	138	± 34 (89–195)
CH:VH	0.43	± 0.10	0.45	± 0.13
Total height μm	582	± 55 (482–667)	438	± 72 (256–577)
Villous width μm	130	± 34 (109–154)	153	± 22 (111–219)
Mitotic index	0.63	± 0.28	0.34	± 0.26

3.3 Epithelial morphology

The villi, which often have a wavy or scalloped outline, are for the most part clothed by tall regular absorptive epithelial cells with a discernible brush border – the 'enterocytes' (Figs. 3.6 and 3.7). The ovoid nuclei of these cells are orientated at right angles to the basement membrane, occupy a fairly constant position closer to the base than the apex of the cell. The enterocytes measure between 30 and 40 μm in height. In many biopsies the epithelial cells appear to be separated by clear spaces (so called Gruenhagen-Mazzanini spaces); this may be due to intercellular oedema, or might perhaps be artefactual. There is, however, some evidence that the extent of these lateral and basal intercellular spaces can be correlated with the absorption of water, as shown by comparisons of experimental *in vivo* and *in vitro* studies (Melligott *et al.*, 1975).

Fig. 3.3 Scanning micrograph of human intestinal biopsy showing a lower power view of the area adjacent to that shown in Fig. 3.1(b). Note the range of villous morphology, from finger-shaped through leaf-shaped to occasional short ridges. Scanning micrograph by courtesy of Dr K. E. Carr.

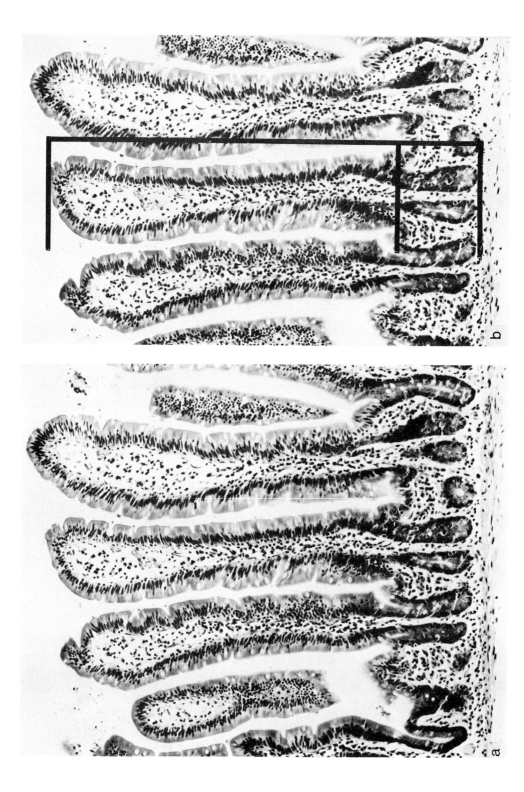

The principal site of absorption is at the tip of the villus, where the cells are most mature and where these spaces are most prominent. A similar correlation between structure and function is encountered in the gall-bladder epithelium, where the absorptive role is equally important. Interspersed between the enterocytes are mucin-secreting goblet cells and occasional endocrine cells. Goblet cells tend to be sparse in the jejunum, but are much more numerous in the distal part of the small intestine.

If a careful examination is made of the epithelial layer, many basally situated small round intercalated nuclei can be seen, which do not belong to true epithelial cells. These are the nuclei of intra-epithelial lymphocytes, which may account for anything up to 30 per cent of the total cell population of the epithelial layer (Ferguson and Murray, 1971). The lymphoid cells appear to enter and leave the epithelium by crossing the basal lamina (Fig. 3.12). They are seemingly involved in the recognition of antigenic stimuli from the luminal contents and in the mounting of appropriate defensive responses. The numbers of intra-epithelial lymphocytes are greatly increased in many intestinal abnormalities, in particular in coeliac disease.

Two other cell types have only recently been recognized in the small intestinal mucosa. The M cell (Owen and Jones, 1974), probably a variant of the enterocyte, occurs in the epithelial layer overlying the lymphoid follicles of Peyer's Patches, and in the appendix. The free surface of this cell does not have the usual enterocyte microvilli, but instead displays low surface convolutions or microfolds (Fig. 3.8), which contrast sharply with the surrounding absorptive cell surfaces. The M cell has a uniquely close relationship with lymphoid cells. Lymphocytes gather in groups, in little pockets surrounded by M cell cytoplasm, separated from the lumen of the gut by an attenuated shell of M cell surface (Fig. 3.10). The lymphocytes do not gain direct access to the lumen, because intercellular adhesion between M cells and enterocytes is maintained, but there is evidence that the M cell selectively picks up macromolecular substances from the lumen and passes them to the lymphocytes (Owen, 1977). These curious cells may,

---

Fig. 3.4 (a) Normal jejunal mucosa, temperate climate. The functional entero-cyte compartment consists of tall slender villi occupying most of the total mucosal height; while the generative epithelium of the crypts accounts for a much smaller proportion. The orientation of this biopsy is regarded as satisfactory since the crypts are visible throughout their entire length. HE × 180.
(b) The normal jejunal mucosa with the principal mucosal compartments outlined diagrammatically. The dividing line between the villous compartment and the crypt compartment is drawn at the point where the villous epithelium curves on to the horizontal plane. HE × 180.

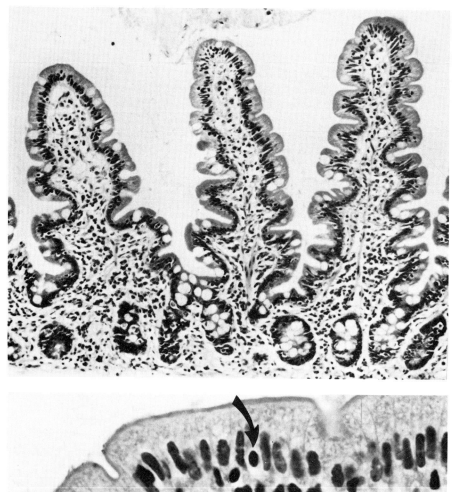

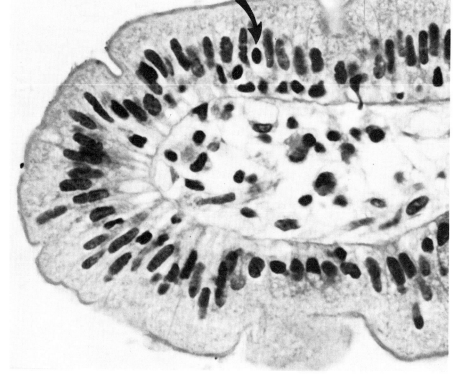

therefore, act as part of the afferent loops of certain immune responses of the intestinal mucosa.

A second cell type recently recognized in the intestine is the tuft cell, (Isomäki, 1973) which has been described in many other mucosal surfaces under various names (Nabeyama and Leblond, 1974). The tuft cell has a distinctive tuft of elongated, thickened microvilli, which extend into the lumen well beyond the level of the surrounding enterocytes (Figs. 3.9 and 3.11). These microvilli have prominent filamentous

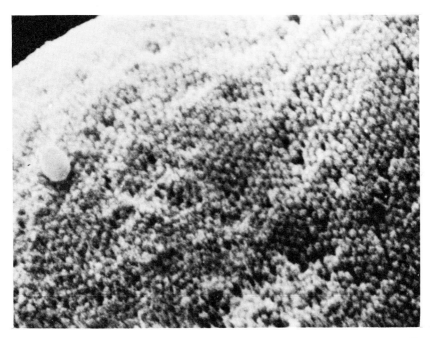

Fig. 3.7 Scanning electron micrograph showing intestinal microvilli. Microvilli are not always as clearly seen as this, their visualization depending partly on the presence of mucus, and perhaps on the state of preservation of the fuzzy coat. Micrograph by courtesy of Dr K. E. Carr.

Fig. 3.5 Normal jejunal mucosa, tropical climate. The villi are broader and shorter than their temperate counterparts (Fig. 3.4) although the crypt:villus ratio is similar. HE × 180.

Fig. 3.6 Normal enterocytes. The cell nuclei are regularly orientated at right angles to the basement membrane. Note the presence of the occasional intra-epithelial lymphocyte (arrowed). In the underlying lamina propria of the villous extremity there is a sparse leucocytic infiltrate consisting mainly of plasma cells and histiocytes. HE × 820.

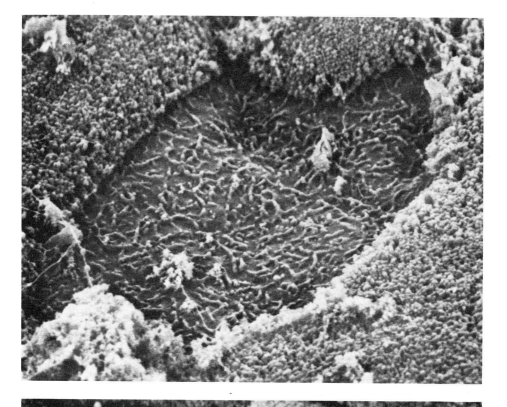

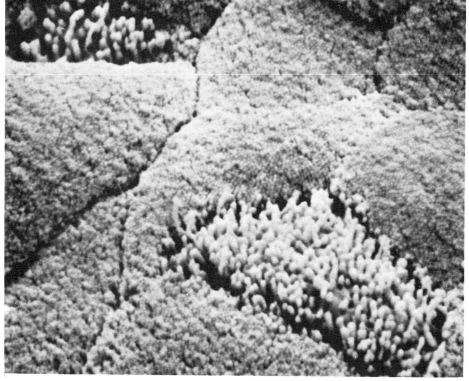

cores which run deep into the apical cytoplasm and twist around the organelles, amongst which there are some apparent pinocytotic vesicles. The presence of tuft cells in the stomach, colon, biliary tract and airways indicates some general mucosal function not specific to the intestine. Perhaps these cells have some as yet unrecognized receptor function in relation to the luminal environment. An unusual carcinoid like tumour of the small intestine recently described by Carstens *et al.* (1976) might possibly represent the neoplastic counterpart of this cell line.

The crypts of Lieberkuhn have a different cellular pattern (Trier and Rubin, 1965). The predominant cell type is the 'enteroblast', the precursor of the enterocyte, in varying stages of maturation. These cells frequently exhibit mitotic activity and occupy the middle or upper parts of the crypts; they show greater cytoplasmic basophilia and less well-developed enzyme systems than their mature counterparts on the villous surface (Padykula *et al.*, 1961). Varying numbers of goblet cells also form part of the epithelial lining of the crypts.

A distinctive feature of the basal parts of the crypts is the presence of Paneth cells, which are characterized by the possession of coarse eosinophilic cytoplasmic granules occupying the supranuclear portion of the cell. Paneth cells are only rarely found on the villous surface except in some inflammatory states; their function is still uncertain, but some clues have recently emerged. For example, it now appears that the Paneth cell granules contain lysozyme. In the rodent, Paneth cells have been shown to ingest organisms of different kinds from the crypt lumen (Erlandsen and Chase, 1972a, b), and immunoglobulins have been detected by some workers within these cells. (Rodning *et al.*, 1976). Perhaps, therefore, the Paneth cell may play some part in the regulation of the intestinal microflora. Distinctive ultrastructural abnormalities of Paneth cells have recently been reported in association with acrodermatitis enteropathica (Bohane *et al.*, 1977), in which zinc deficiency has now been identified; Paneth cells are known to concentrate zinc to a greater degree than almost any other cell in the body. The functional significance of this remains to be clarified.

Fig. 3.8 Scanning micrograph showing the contrast between the surface of the intestinal M cell and the surrounding enterocytes. The normal enterocyte microvilli can be clearly seen, but the surface of the M cell is covered by low convoluted ridges or microfolds. Micrograph by courtesy of Dr R. L. Owen.
Fig. 3.9 Scanning micrograph showing the contrast between the prominent microvilli of two tuft cells and the smaller conventional microvilli of the surrounding enterocytes. The tuft cell microvilli protrude further from the surface and are thicker and more prominent than those on the neighbouring cells. Micrograph by courtesy of Dr R. L. Owen.

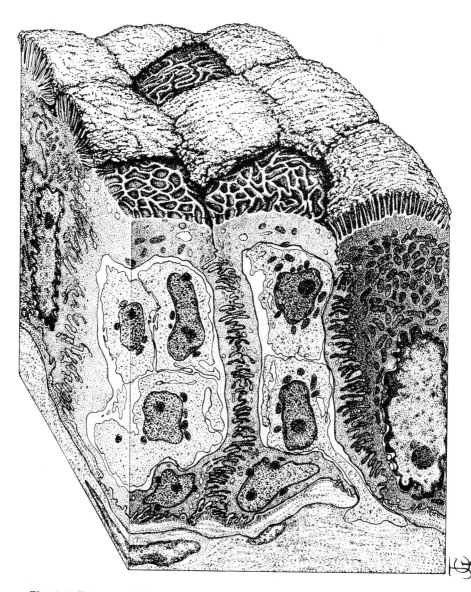

Fig. 3.10 Diagram of the relationship between intestinal M cells and lymphocytes. The lymphoid cells occupy pockets enclosed by M cell cytoplasm. A thin
shell of M cell cytoplasm separates the lymphoid cells from the intestinal
lumen. Diagram by courtesy of Dr R. L. Owen.

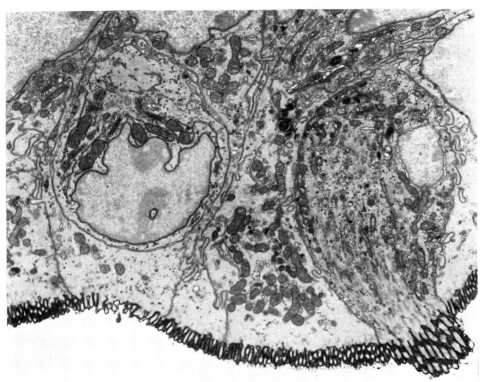

Fig. 3.11 Transmission electron micrograph showing the apical portion of an intestinal tuft cell with adjacent enterocytes. Note the prominence of the tuft of microvilli which projects far beyond the level of the surfaces of adjacent enterocytes. Micrograph by courtesy of Dr R. L. Owen (1977).

Endocrine cells are more numerous in the basal parts of the crypts than elsewhere; they can generally be identified in HE-stained sections by their pyramidal shape and by the presence of fine infranuclear cytoplasmic granules of brick-red colour. In some instances the nuclei typically appear to be surrounded by a clear cytoplasmic zone. The argentaffin cells, the most numerous of the endocrine group, are so named because of the capacity of their cytoplasmic granules to form metallic silver from silver salts; this is related to the presence of 5-hydroxytryptamine. They are the most well-known members of a larger class of polypeptide hormone-producing cells, claimed as part of the APUD cell system (Pearse *et al.*, 1977), which are found scattered within all epithelial surfaces of endodermal origin. Members of the APUD system apart from the argentaffin cells usually lack the capacity to form metallic silver from silver salts, although some can do so in the presence of external reducing agents, a property termed argyrophilia. More accurate identification of these cell types can be achieved by ultrastructural or immunohistochemical techniques.

3.4 Lamina propria mucosae

This consists of a framework of fibroblasts and argyrophilic 'reticulin' enclosing blood vessels, lymphatics, smooth muscle fibres and connective tissue cells. Leucocytes are also invariably present, although their numbers vary widely. Four types of leucocyte are constantly found.

(a) *Lymphoid cells* In about 20 per cent of normal biopsies solitary lymphoid follicles are seen in the lamina propria or in the submucosa in close apposition to the lamina muscularis mucosae. Germinal centres are not often visible in adult biopsies but are more conspicuous in childhood. A diffuse infiltrate of small lymphocytes can be detected apart from discrete follicles, usually in the deeper layers of the lamina propria. The lymphocytes within the epithelial lining (intra-epithelial lymphocytes or theliolymphocytes) are, however, much more conspicuous and, as previously mentioned, may account for up to 30 per cent of the nuclei in the epithelial surface (Fig. 3.5, 3.6 and 3.12).

(b) *Plasma cells* These are invariably present and diffusely distributed throughout the lamina propria. Apart from lymphoid follicles, plasma cells are more numerous than lymphocytes, but are never found in the epithelial layer. Russell bodies are occasionally seen.

(c) *Eosinophils* Another invariable component of the jejunal mucosa, eosinophils, may be sparse in the lamina propria. Only on rare occasions are these cells seen in the epithelial surface. Neutrophils are rarely if ever seen in biopsies under normal conditions unless blood has been extravasated as a result of biopsy trauma. Mast cells likewise are only rarely found in the intestinal mucosa (Scott *et al.*, 1975).

(d) *Histiocytes* Histiocytes are most easily found at the villous extremity in close relationship to the subepithelial reticulin network (Fig. 3.6). Sometimes they contain flecks of haematoxyphilic material, presumably representing nuclear debris, and deposits of unidentified pigment. The presence of haemosiderin in these cells or in the epithelium cannot be regarded as normal in temperate biopsies (Section 4.1.3); it is, however, quite commonly seen in healthy tropical residents, and can probably be attributed to the imbibition of liquids with a high iron content.

Recently, histometric methods have been used to quantitate the individual cellular components of the leucocytic infiltrate (Holmes *et al.*, 1973). Although mainly used to assess pathological alteration, it

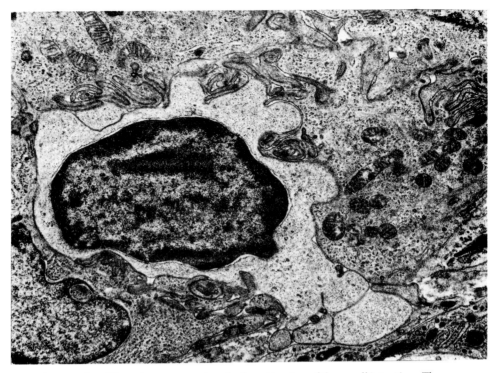

Fig. 3.12 Small lymphocyte crossing the basal lamina of the small intestine. The nucleus of the lymphocyte and most of its cytoplasm lies between the basal portions of the columnar enterocytes. A small tail of lymphocyte cytoplasm protrudes into the lamina propria and lies in contact with a macrophage. There is a gap in the basal lamina at the point where the lymphocyte is crossing the junction between epithelium and lamina propria. Notice the absence of cytoplasmic differentiation within the lymphocyte.

may be possible by these methods to establish the limits of the normal leucocytic infiltrate.

3.5 The dynamic basis of mucosal structure

Under normal conditions the mature absorptive epithelial cell or 'enterocyte' in man is thought to have a life span or cell cycle time of just over 2 days (Watson and Wright, 1974). In other words, almost half of the enterocyte population has to be replaced every day. New enterocytes are derived from the mitotic division of undifferentiated stem cells (enteroblasts) located in middle or uppers parts of the crypts of Lieberkühn. The developing cells emerge from the crypts and ascend the villous surface in step-ladder fashion, displacing the more mature cells which are ultimately extruded from the villous extremity (Potten and Allen, 1977). Normal mucosal architecture depends to a large extent upon the integrity of this process of replication. Clinical and experimental studies have shown, for example, that when the entero-blasts are destroyed by ionising radiation or cytotoxic drugs, the production of enterocytes ceases and the villi collapse (see Clark and Harland, 1963 and Wiernik, 1966). A similar phenomenon comes about when the life span of the enterocyte is seriously curtailed, as appears to be the case in coeliac disease (Section 4.2.1); should the crypt entero-blasts fail to meet the increased demand for new cells which results, a stable state can only be reached through acceptance of a greatly reduced enterocyte population, which can only be achieved through villous collapse.

While direct measurement of enterocyte life span may have clinical value, it is seldom feasible. Radioisotopic methods have been employed in exceptional circumstances and DNA measurements from luminal perfusion experiments can provide quantitative data on cell shedding. An indirect assessment of life span can be made from calculation of the ratio between crypt height (CH) and villous height (VH) which approximates to the ratio between the enteroblast population and the functional enterocyte population. As has been mentioned (Section 3.2) the CH:VH ratio rarely exceeds 0.6 in normal individuals, regardless of the climatic conditions and is usually between 0.4 and 0.5. The percentage of epithelial cells in mitotic division (the mitotic index) may be a further reflection of enterocyte life span, although this difficult and laborious measurement is unlikely to be widely applied in routine diagnostic pathology.

3.6 Conclusions

The normal intestinal mucosa can only be defined histologically as the appearance of the mucosa in apparently normal individuals. It has become only too evident that this is subject to considerable variability, particularly with regard to mucosal architecture. The 'temperate' and 'tropical' versions of normality probably represent the ends of a spectrum, and it seems likely that there are intermediate patterns corresponding to intermediate climatic conditions and possibly to dietary variations. It cannot be over-emphasized that mucosal abnormality must always be assessed against the background of the normal variation in any particular community.

There are, however, two features which appear to be characteristic of the normal intestinal mucosa, regardless of geographical or individual factors. First, the villous height and morphology, reflecting the mature enterocyte population, is appropriate to the climatic conditions; and secondly, enterocyte production balances cell loss with a CH:VH ratio which is around 0.4 and 0.5 and seldom exceeds 0.6, this being considered as the morphological expression of a normal enterocyte life span.

References

Anderson, J. H. and Taylor, A. B. (1973), Scanning and transmission electron microscopic studies of jejunal microvilli of the rat, hamster and dog. *J. Morph.*, **141**, 281–291.

Bohane, T. D., Cutz, E., Hamilton, J. R. and Gall, D. G. (1977), Acrodermatitis enteropathica, zinc and the Paneth cell. A case report with family studies. *Gastroenterology*, **73**, 587–592.

Booth, C. C., Stewart, J. S., Holmes, R. and Brackenburg, W. (1962), Dissecting microscope appearance of intestinal mucosa. In *Ciba Foundation Study Group No. 14: Intestinal Biopsy*, (Ed. Wolstenholme, G. E. W. and Cameron, M. P.), pp. 2–23. Churchill, London.

Carstens, P. H. B., Broghamer, W. L. and Hire, D. (1976), Malignant fibrillocaveolated cell carcinoma of the human intestinal tract. *Human Pathol.*, **7**, 505–517.

Clark, P. A. and Harland, W. A. (1963), Experimental malabsorption with jejunal atrophy induced by colchicine. *Br. J. exp. Path.*, **44**, 520–523.

Erlandsen, S. L. and Chase, D. G. (1972a), Paneth cell function: phagocytosis and intracellular digestion of intestinal microorganisms. I. *Hexamita muris*. *J. Ultrastruct. Res.*, **41**, 296–318.

Erlandsen, S. L. and Chase, D. G. (1972b), Paneth cell function: phagocytosis and intracellular digestion of intestinal microorganisms. II. Spiral microorganisms. *J. Ultrastruct. Res.*, **41**, 319–333.

Ferguson, A. and Murray, D. (1971), Quantitation of intraepithelial lymphocytes in human jejunum. *Gut*, **12**, 988–994.

Holmes, G. K. T., Asquith, P., Stokes, P. J. and Cooke, W. T. (1973), Cellular infiltrate of jejunal biopsies in adult coeliac disease in relation to gluten withdrawal. *Gut*, **14**, 429. (Abstract)

Isomäki, A. M. (1973), A new cell type (tuft cell) in the gastrointestinal mucosa of the rat. A transmission and scanning electron microscopic study. *Acta path. microbiol. Scand. (A)*: Suppl. 240, 1–35.

Lee, F. D. (1970), *The intestinal mucosa in health and disease*. M.D. Thesis, University of Dundee.

Lindenbaum, J., Kent, T. H. and Sprinz, H. (1966), Malabsorption and jejunitis in American Peace Corps Volunteers in Pakistan. *Ann. intern. Med.*, 1201–1209.

Mathan, M., Mathan, V. I. and Baker, S. J. (1975), An electron microscopic study of jejunal mucosal morphology in control subjects and in patients with tropical sprue in Southern India. *Gastroenterology*, **68**, 17–32.

Melligott, T. F., Beck, I. T., Dinda, P. K. and Thompson, S. (1975), Correlation of structural changes at different levels of the jejunal villus with positive net water transport *in vivo* and *in vitro*. *Can. J. Physiol. Pharmacol.*, **53**, 439–450.

Nabeyama, A. and Leblond, C. P. (1974), 'Caveolated Cells' characterized by deep surface invaginations and abundant filaments in mouse gastro-intestinal epithelia. *Am. J. Anat.*, **140**, 147–166.

Owen, R. L. (1977), Sequential uptake of horseradish peroxidase by lymphoid follicle epithelium of Peyer's patches in the normal unobstructed mouse intestine: an ultrastructural study. *Gastroenterology*, **72**, 440–451.

Owen, R. L. and Brandborg, L. L. (1977), Jejunal morphologic consequences of vegetarian diet in humans. *Gastroenterology*, **72**, A-88/1111.

Owen, R. L. and Jones, A. L. (1974), Epithelial cell specialization within human Peyer's patches: an ultrastructural study of intestinal lymphoid follicles. *Gastroenterology*, **66**, 189–203.

Padykula, H. A., Strauss, E. W., Ladman, A. J. and Gardner, F. H. (1961), A morphologic and histochemical analysis of the human jejunal epithelium in nontropical sprue. *Gastroenterology*, **40**, 735–765.

Pearse, A. G. E., Polak, J. M. and Bloom, S. R. (1977), The newer gut hormones. Cellular sources, physiology, pathology and clinical aspects. *Gastroenterology*, **72**, 746–761.

Potten, C. S. and Allen, T. D. (1977), Ultrastructure of cell loss in the intestinal mucosa. *J. Ultrastruct. Res.*, **60**, 272–277.

Rodning, C. B., Wilson, I. D. and Erlandsen, S. L. (1976), Immunoglobulins within human small intestinal Paneth cells. *Lancet*, **1**, 984–987.

Scott, B. B., Hardy, G. J. and Losowsky, M. S. (1975), Involvement of the small intestine in systemic mast cell disease. *Gut*, **16**, 918–924.

Stewart, J. S., Pollock, D. J., Hoffbrand, A. V., Mollin, D. L. and Booth, C. C. (1967), A study of proximal and distal intestinal structure and absorptive function in idiopathic steatorrhoea. *Q. J. Med.*, **36**, 425–444.

Trier, J. S. and Rubin, C. E. (1965), Electron microscopy of the small intestine. A review. *Gastroenterology*, **49**, 574–603.

Watson, A. J. and Wright, N. A. (1974), Morphology and cell kinetics of the jejunal mucosa in untreated patients. In *Clinics in Gastroenterology*, 3, No. 1 *(Coeliac disease)*, p. 20. Saunders, London.

Wiernik, G. (1966), Changes in the villous pattern of the human jejunum associated with heavy radiation damage. *Gut*, **7**, 149–153.

4 The assessment of intestinal abnormality

4.1 General examination of the biopsy

The pathologist must be alert to the clinical setting of the intestinal biopsy, which may focus attention on some special aspect. The age of the patient and the detailed medical history will often narrow the diagnostic choice. For example, amyloidosis could easily be over-looked if a history of rheumatoid arthritis is not known. Preparations for special techniques such as electron microscopy or enzyme analysis must be made in advance of the biopsy. If dissecting microscopy is planned, the biopsy should be examined under saline immediately after removal from the capsule (see Section 2.2). A simple grading system for recording the results of dissecting microscopy is provided in Table 2.1.

A systematic approach is essential for histological assessment. The best orientated section is selected from at least three histological levels for the preliminary evaluation of mucosal architecture. The main pathological villous patterns (Section 4.2) are summarized in Table 4.1. These findings can then be related to the dissecting microscope appearance.

After this general assessment, the different anatomical parts of the biopsy should be carefully studied in order.

4.1.1 Luminal changes

Examination of the intestinal lumen for parasites should never be omitted, regardless of the geographical origin of the biopsy. In Britain, the protozoon *Giardia lamblia* is the commonest parasitic infestation. It may cause malabsorption, especially in children and young adults,

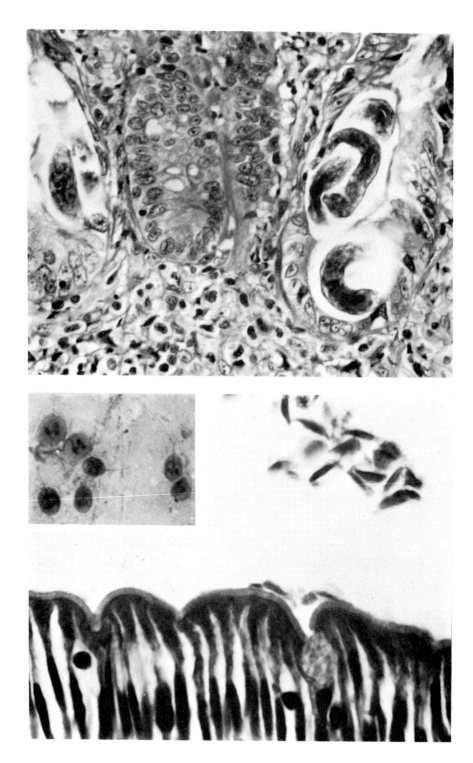

and is common in certain types of immune deficiency in adults. The parasite is easily seen in histological sections, although Giemsa stained smears freshly prepared from the mucus adhering to the biopsy greatly increase the chance of detection (Fig. 4.2). The electron microscopic appearances (Figs. 4.3 and 4.4.) are highly characteristic (Erlandsen and Chase, 1974; Klima *et al.*, 1977). Symptoms may be caused by mechanical occlusion of a large part of the enterocyte surface. Less commonly, hookworm disease or intestinal capillariasis can be detected by random intestinal biopsy, the organisms being found mainly within crypt lumina (Fig. 4.1).

4.1.2 *Epithelial changes*

The epithelial surface must next be examined. The height, regularity, cytoplasmic appearance, nuclear morphology and nuclear polarity of the enterocytes should be carefully assessed, and an estimate made of the number of goblet cells and intra-epithelial lymphocytes (3.4). In coeliac disease for example, the various cytological changes affecting the enterocytes are most marked at the villous extremity and precede any change in villous architecture (Figs. 4.5 and 4.6). Booth (1968) has contrasted these 'microcytic' changes with the 'macrocytic' enterocytes sometimes seen in B12 and folate deficiency (see also Foroozan and Trier, 1967). In abetalipoproteinaemia, a rare inherited condition, vacuolation of the enterocytes is shown by frozen sections to be due to the presence of neutral fat (Fig. 4.7). On electron microscopy, the brush border is normal but chylomicrons are absent from the basal intercellular spaces. The defect here is one of fat transport rather than fat absorption (Fig. 4.8).

Stainable iron within enterocytes is uncommon in developed countries, and usually indicates haemochromatosis (Astaldi *et al.*, 1966) or transfusional haemosiderosis (Cappell *et al.*, 1957). In certain parts of Africa this finding is much more common, and is attributable to excess of iron intake.

Metaplastic changes involve the replacement of enterocytes by cells showing a different differentiation pattern. Cells similar to those of the

---

Fig. 4.1 Jejunal biopsy. Vegetative forms of *Necator americanus* are present in the lumen of the crypts. HE × 620.

Fig. 4.2 Jejunal biopsy. Vegetative forms of *Giardia lamblia* are clearly demonstrated in the intestinal lumen and some appear to be attached to the epithelial surface (HE × 1200). The insert (top left) illustrates the appearance of the organisms in a cytological smear of aspirated duodenal secretion stained by the Giemsa method (× 1200).

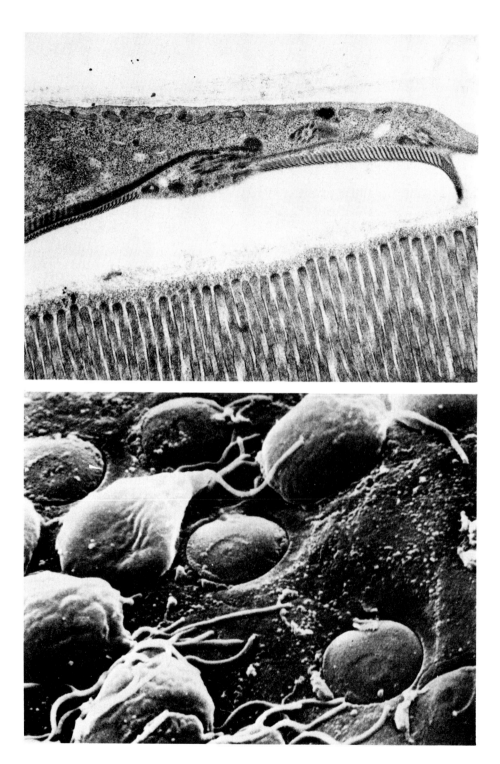

gastric surface layer are common in the duodenum (James, 1964) in relation to high acid levels (Fig. 4.10; Patrick et al., 1974). More distally, pyloric or gastric metaplasia may be more extensive, particularly in association with inflammatory disease.

Minor histological changes may be noted in protein malnutrition in adults and in kwashiorkor in infants (Duque et al., 1975; Brunser et al., 1976). More extensive ultrastructural changes have now been described in these conditions. These changes include shortening, branching and fusion of microvilli and increase in the lysosome population of the enterocytes. Ultrastructural studies have also shown changes in patients undergoing prolonged fasting, in patients with alcoholic cirrhosis, and in patients subjected to controlled dietary carbohydrate substitution by alcohol (Rubin et al., 1972). Subcellular changes have been shown in enterocyte mitochondria following exposure to staphylococcal enterotoxin (Merril and Sprinz, 1968) but ultrastructural damage is not seen in the case of cholera toxin (Norris and Majno, 1968), which acts by stimulating existing physiological secretory mechanisms.

Changes in the crypts of Lieberkühn are more difficult to assess. The stem cell population is particularly susceptible to irradiation, which produces focal cytoplasmic damage. Sufficient dosage will halt mitotic activity with subsequent degradation of the mucosal lining. 'Cytomegalic' changes have been reported in some cases of vitamin B12 and folic acid deficiency (Foroozan and Trier, 1967). In folic acid deficiency such changes have been found regularly only in children (Davidson and Townley, 1977). Such deficiencies might perhaps be responsible for cytomegalic changes in occasional cases of adult coeliac disease (Ten Thije, 1963) and in some fatal cases of kwashiorkor (Fig. 4.12).

The Paneth cells may be reduced in number in coeliac disease (Ward et al., 1976) and Kwashiorkor (Trowell et al., 1954). These changes are

---

Fig. 4.3 Transmission electron micrograph showing intestinal microvilli with the overlying fuzzy coat. Close to the surface lies part of the parasite Giardia lamblia. The complex internal organization of the parasite is seen, and the elaborate striation of the undersurface of the parasite is obvious. Several obliquely sectioned centrioles are noted. These are the basal bodies of the flagella of the parasite.

Fig. 4.4 Scanning electron micrograph of Giardia lamblia parasites on the surface of the intestinal mucosa. The tadpole-shaped parasites and their flagella are clearly seen. Several parasites have become detached during processing for scanning electron microscopy. The impressions left by these parasites on the mucosal surface appear as rounded, disc-shaped areas. Micrograph by courtesy of Dr S. L. Erlandsen.

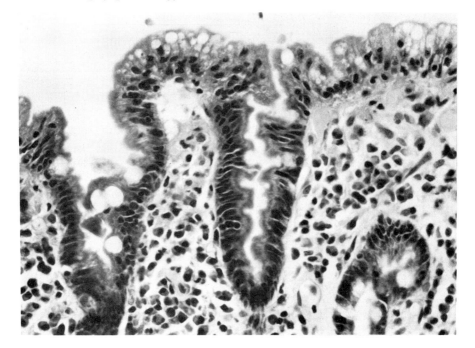

Fig. 4.5 Coeliac disease. The enterocytes on the mucosal surface show irregularity of shape and disturbed polarity. There is also an increase in the number of intra-epithelial lymphocytes, and an augmented plasma-cell infiltrate in the lamina propria. HE × 450.

reversible on treatment, although in some cases of supposed coeliac disease an exceptionally marked deficiency of Paneth cells may be associated with the poor response to therapy (Pink and Creamer, 1967). On the other hand, Paneth cells are unusually prominent in some cases of Crohn's disease. This Paneth cell response to chronic inflammation is similar to that seen in the colon in chronic inflammatory disease, particularly ulcerative colitis (Watson and Roy, 1960). The presence of Paneth cell abnormalities in acrodermatitis enteropathica is mentioned elsewhere (Section 5.3).

The responses of the intestinal endocrine cells in disease are not well documented. Increased numbers of endocrine cells reported in coeliac disease and tropical sprue may be a consequence of the increased production of enterocytes which characterizes both conditions. Goblet cells may also be increased in coeliac disease (Stewart *et al.*, 1967).

The crypts of Lieberkühn may be affected by 'crypt abscesses'. This well-recognized feature of colonic disease is also found in the stomach and small intestine. It is probably a non-specific manifestation of epithelial damage, initiated by focal breakdown in the crypt epithelium (Fig. 4.13). Emigrating neutrophils, accompanied as a rule by red cells and mucus, may initially escape from the crypt, but are ultimately blocked by the formation of adhesions between damaged epithelial cells at the crypt mouth (Fig. 4.14). The characteristic crypt distension then results (Fig. 4.15). The distended crypt finally ruptures, usually into the intestinal lumen. Probably most forms of ulceration arise in this way; it is notable that the crypt abscess is commonly associated with the localized hypertrophic villous pattern which is also a pre-ulcerative disturbance (Section 4.2.2). The crypt abscess has no specific connotation, but a specific cause for the lesion can sometimes be identified. In Crohn's disease it may result from erosion of a granulomatous focus through the crypt epithelium (Fig. 4.16).

A second important pathological change in the intestinal crypt is metaplasia. This usually involves an alteration towards gastric-type epithelium. Metaplasia is an acquired form of heterotopia which develops as a consequence of chronic irritation. It must be clearly distinguished from congenital heterotopia such as may be found in Meckel's diverticulum. Gastric metaplasia in the small bowel, initially associated exclusively with Crohn's disease (Liber, 1951), can in fact occur in any form of chronic intestinal inflammation, especially where there is recurrent epithelial damage (Lee, 1964). Like the crypt abscess, it commonly accompanies the localized hypertrophic villous pattern (Section 4.2.2). Metaplasia first affects the crypts, which change from simple tubes to branching glands (Fig. 4.17). The lining cells contain neutral mucin compared with the normal mucicarminophilic goblet cells of the crypts. With their basally situated nuclei (Fig. 7.4), these cells closely resemble the glandular epithelium of the pyloric antrum. In florid cases, the villous epithelium is replaced by surface epithelium similar to that of the stomach (Fig. 4.18). The term pyloric metaplasia describes this resemblance to antral mucosa. The more comprehensive term 'gastric metaplasia' may be more appropriate since parietal and zymogenic cells may be detected (Yokoyama et al., 1977; Fig. 4.19).

4.1.3 Changes in the lamina propria

Changes in the leukocyte population are the most important of the pathological alterations of the lamina propria. By far the most common is the non-specific response, simply an exaggeration of the normal leukocytic infiltrate (Section 3.4) with increased numbers of plasma cells. In more severe disease the leukocyte changes may be associated with fibrosis (Fig. 4.20) or collagen formation (Figs. 4.40 and 4.42) in the

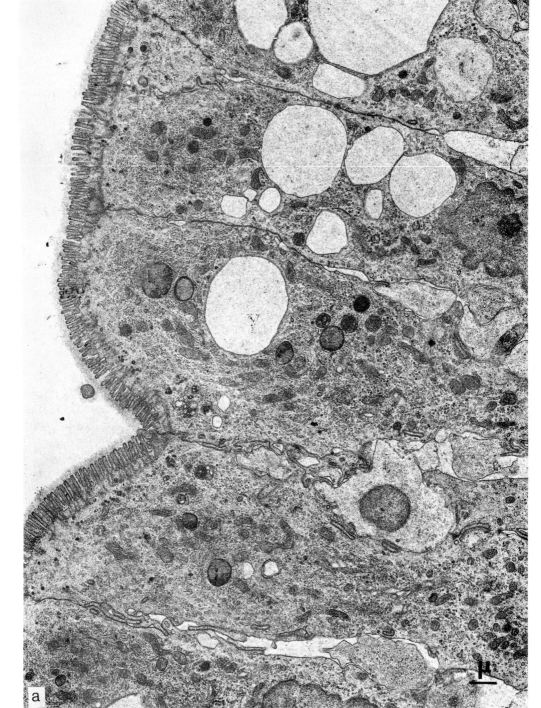

a

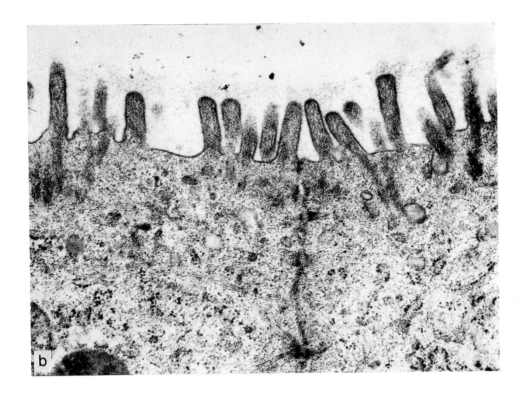

Fig. 4.6(a) Transmission electron micrograph of intestinal mucosa in a case of coeliac disease. The abnormality is not of the severest degree, since the intestinal microvilli remain reasonably well-preserved. They are, however, shorter than normal, while the underlying cytoplasm shows various abnormalities. These include the presence of vacuoles, increased numbers of lysosome-like bodies, and increased numbers of interstitial lymphocytes.

(b) Intestinal microvilli in a more severe case of coeliac disease. Note the shortening, sparseness, and variable orientation of the remaining microvilli.

lamina propria. This is seldom prominent in coeliac disease, but is more commonly associated with the hypertrophic villous pattern invariably found near gross ulcerative lesions, regardless of their cause (Section 4.2.2). An unusual predominance of lymphocytes in the lamina propria should always raise the suspicion of lymphoid neoplasia, especially in association with coeliac disease (Section 5.1). A similar predominance of small lymphocytes may also be seen in Crohn's disease. Increased numbers of neutrophil polymorphs in the

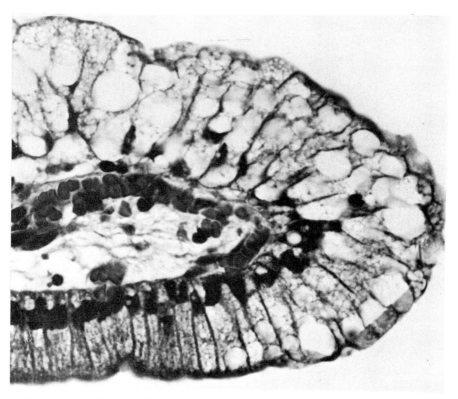

Fig. 4.7 Abetalipoproteinaemia. The enterocytes at the villous extremity show pronounced vacuolation with 'ballooning' of the cytoplasm in some cells. HE × 815.

Fig. 4.8 Transmission electron micrograph of intestinal mucosa in a case of abetalipoproteinaemia. The microvilli of the enterocytes are completely normal, as are the cytoplasmic organelles. The cells however contain substantial amounts of stored lipid material in the form of large round pale droplets. This fatty accumulation reflects the failure of the intestinal mucosa to discharge lipid in the normal fashion as chylomicrons. Micrograph by courtesy of Dr I. A. R. More.

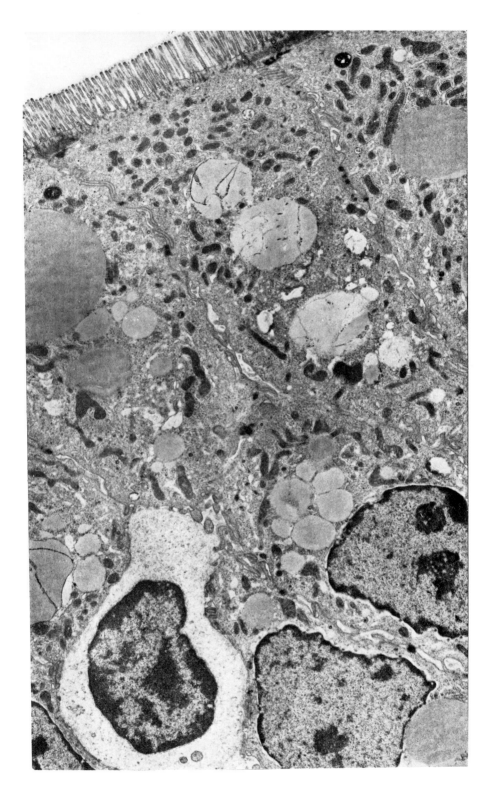

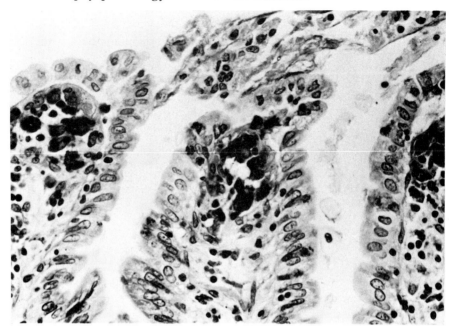

Fig. 4.9 Mucosal haemosiderosis. The histiocytes at the villous extremity contain large quantities of stainable iron. The patient suffered from rheumatoid arthritis with amyloidosis. Perl's prussian blue × 450.

lamina propria may be provoked by epithelial damage no matter how it is produced. In the proximal duodenum, 'active' inflammation such as this probably represents a phase in the evolution or regression of peptic ulceration (Section 8.3, Fig. 4.10). Neutrophil emigration may also be a feature of ischaemic damage to the intestinal mucosa (Fig. 4.21) and is seen in some cases of Whipple's disease. Acute lesions are rarely seen in coeliac disease, but have been provoked in the ileum by experimental gluten challenge (Rubin *et al.*, 1962). Increased numbers of eosinophil polymorphs in the lamina propria are particularly associated with allergic disturbances such as eosinophilic gastroenteritis and allergic gastroenteropathy of childhood. A slight increase has also been observed in tropical sprue, while curiously, parasitic disease only rarely produces a significant mucosal eosinophilia. Atypical lymphoid cells have occasionally been found in viral disease such as infective hepatitis (Conrad *et al.*, 1964) and infectious mononucleosis (Sheehy *et al.*, 1964).

Inflammatory reactions characterized mainly by a histiocytic response are of diagnostic importance. The classical sarcoid granuloma is generally considered to be a manifestation of the delayed hypersensitivity reaction. In this country, Crohn's disease is by far the commonest cause, although the mucosa itself contains sarcoid follicles (Fig. 4.22) only in a minority of cases. Tuberculosis, the only important differential diagnosis, must always be rigorously excluded. Sarcoidosis itself rarely affects the intestinal tract and fungal disease is uncommon. In the tropics granulomas caused by helminthic infestation are occasionally seen: the cause of these is usually seen on histology.

Diffuse or non-follicular histiocytic responses may also be seen. During the intestinal phase of the enteric fevers, the inflamed lymphoid aggregates of the small intestine typically show accumulation of globular histiocytes, many of which contain phagocytosed red cells or nuclear debris (Fig. 4.23). Diffuse histiocytic infiltration may also be seen in viral enteritis such as cytomegalic inclusion body disease (Fig. 4.24). The Warthin-Finkeldey cells sometimes found in the intestine in measles (Fig. 4.25) may also be of histiocytic origin.

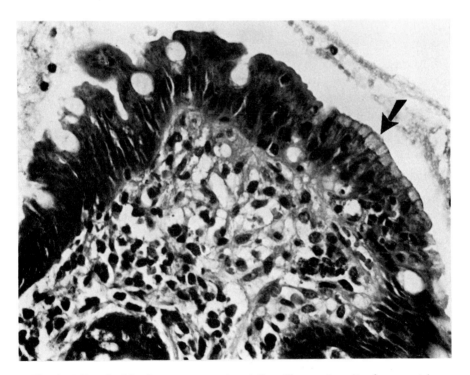

Fig. 4.10 Duodenitis. Some enterocytes at the villous extremity show gastric metaplasia, characterized by the presence of globules of neutral mucin in the luminal aspect of the cytoplasm (arrowed). Others show cytoplasmic basophilia and syncytial tufting. There is also an augmented leucocytic infiltrate in the lamina propria. HE × 450.

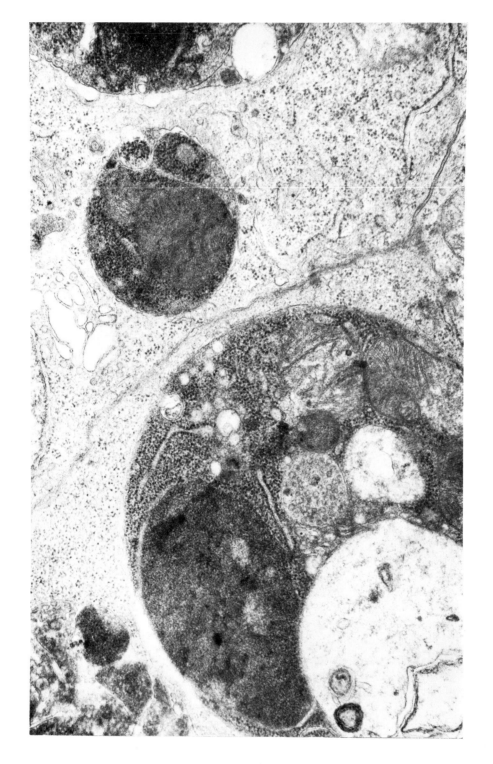

Whipple's disease, an uncommon condition, is characterized by a diffuse histiocytic infiltrate (Maizel *et al.*, 1970). The cells contain PAS positive granules consisting of neutral polysaccharides of presumed bacterial origin (Fig. 4.26). Distinctive rod-shaped organisms, first detected by electron microscopy, are widely spread throughout the lamina propria (Fig. 4.28) and may be seen between epithelial cells. The macrophages engulf these organisms in large phagosomes where they are partially broken down (Fig. 4.29). Residual masses of undigested material remain for substantial periods of time within the macrophage (Fig. 4.27). Similar features may be seen in lymph nodes and in more distant organs. The organisms have not yet been conclusively identified but their occurrence correlates well with clinical findings (Trier *et al.*, 1965; Morningstar, 1975). Malacoplakia, also extremely rare (Ranchod and Kahn, 1972; Sanusi and Tio, 1974), may share some common mechanism with Whipple's disease. Electron microscopy has shown the presence of rod-shaped organisms in this condition as well (Lewin *et al.*, 1974). The laminated and calcified spherical Michaelis-Guttman bodies represent encrustations upon masses of undigested bacterial residues.

Lipid-containing histiocytes or 'lipophages' may occur when lymphatic drainage is obstructed, whether by congenital intestinal lymphangiectasia, or as a result of disease such as jejunal diverticulosis, tuberculosis or tumour. Foamy histiocytes have also been described in chronic granulomatous disease (Ament and Ochs, 1973). Haemosiderin laden histiocytes in the lamina propria, especially at the villous tip, are common in tropical Africa, but uncommon in developed countries. This is usually due to a condition of iron overload as in transfusion haemosiderosis or haemochromatosis. The occurrence of haemosiderosis along with generalized iron depletion in Whipple's disease (Hourihane, 1966) and in rheumatoid arthritis (Lee *et al.*, 1978) may indicate a disturbance of phagocytic function and iron absorption in these conditions.

The leukocyte population of the lamina propria may reflect the immunological status of the patient. Severe generalized hypogammaglobulinaemia, whether congenital or acquired, is usually accompanied by a pronounced reduction in plasma cells (Fig. 4.30). Large lymphoid aggregates with prominent germinal centres are found in some immuno-deficiency states (Fig. 4.31) although in classical sex-

---

Fig. 4.11 Crypt cells from mouse intestinal mucosa following radiation injury. Several large round inclusions are seen within the cells. These contain fragments of still recognizable cytoplasmic organelles. Within these inclusions, the damaged fragments of cytoplasm are digested by lysosomal enzymes.

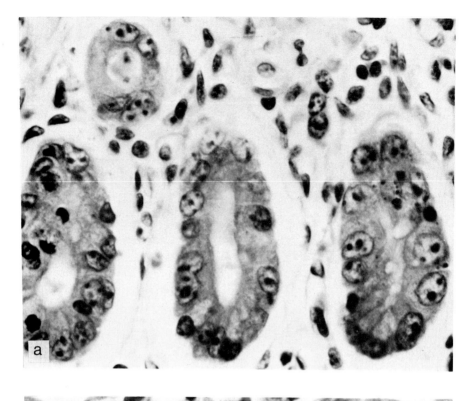

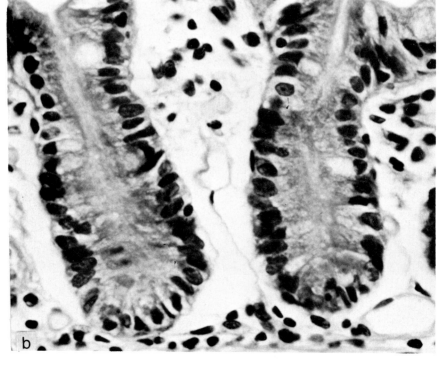

linked hypogammaglobulinaemia germinal centres are notably absent. The presence of unusual intestinal infections in adult life, such as cytomegalic inclusion body disease (Fig. 4.24) or giardiasis (Fig. 4.30), may also raise suspicion of an immunodeficient state.

Apart from the fibrosis which accompanies inflammatory disease, abnormalities of the connective tissues are uncommon. Dilatation of mucosal lymphatic channels, quite a common isolated finding in normal biopsies, may, if extensive, raise the possibility of lymphatic obstruction. The presence of lipophages may have a similar significance. Mucosal lymphangiectasia may also be a feature of Crohn's disease (Fig. 4.32). Amyloidosis (Fig. 4.33) is the most important vascular lesion in the lamina propria. In several cases, the epithelial basement membranes may be affected as well as the vessel walls. Masses of amorphous hyaline material, probably IgM immunoglobulin, have been found in the lamina propria in some cases of Waldenstrom's macroglobulinaemia (Pruzanski et al., 1973; Fig. 4.34). Finally, the lamina muscularis mucosae often included in the biopsy, may occasionally show the presence of paranuclear lipofuscin pigmentation (Fig. 4.35). This may provide useful evidence of malabsorption. (Section 5.1) Lipofuscin is best seen in sections stained by the PAS or long acid-fast techniques.

4.1.4 *Submucosa*

Large areas of submucosa are not usually present in a peroral intestinal biopsy, but careful study should be made of any deep tissue seen. In Crohn's disease, involvement of the submucosa by the granulomatous inflammation is characteristic. Amyloid deposition (Fig. 4.33) and vasculitis, such as in polyarteritis nodosa or rheumatoid arthritis, are more readily detected in the submucosa than elsewhere. Submucosal oedema and eosinophil polymorph infiltration is characteristic of one important variant of the allergic condition eosinophilic gastroenteritis (Fig. 4.36).

4.2 The classification of villous abnormality

A universally acceptable system for classifying villous abnormality is not at present available. There are several reasons for this, such as lack

---

Fig. 4.12(a) Kwashiorkor. In this fatal case the enteroblasts in the crypts of Lieberkühn show pronounced cytomegalic change in the nuclei (cf. Fig. 4.12b) HE × 820.
(b) Normal crypts of Lieberkühn. Note the size and regularity of the enteroblastic nuclei when compared with those in (a) HE × 820.

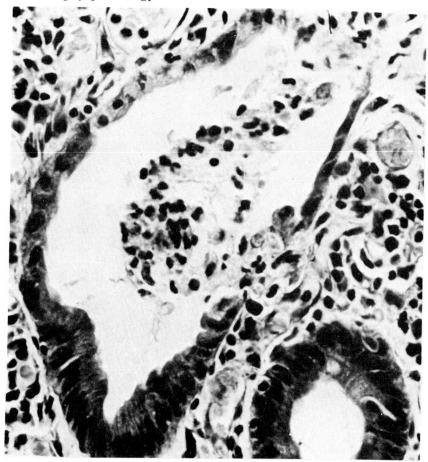

Fig. 4.13 Early crypt abscess. There is micro-ulceration of the crypt epithelium with emigration of neutrophil polymorphs into the crypt lumen. HE × 525.

of agreement on terminology and difficulties in defining the limits of normal variation. Research workers in this field have thus tended to adopt individualized methods of assessment.

In the early years following the introduction of intestinal biopsy, the classification of villous abnormality was based exclusively on light microscopy of histological sections. Thus Shiner and Doniach (1960), employing histological measurement, recognized two types of pathological abnormality which they designated partial villous atrophy (P.V.A.) and subtotal villous atrophy (S.V.A.). Rubin and his colleagues (1960) preferred to avoid the term 'atrophy', initially introduced by Paulley (1954), and simply described the histological deviation from normality as mild, moderate or severe; while these workers were the first to describe the examination of biopsies under the dissecting microscope, they regard histology as by far the most important procedure in the assessment of biopsies (see also Perera *et al.*, 1975).

Nevertheless, dissecting microscopy became widely used in Britain as a method of grading biopsies, since it was thought that this technique might overcome the problem of histological orientation (Section 2.3) and the variability of villous pattern observed in some biopsies (Booth *et al.*, 1962). The dissecting microscope appearances can, however, be difficult to quantitate, and there is sometimes poor correlation with the histological findings (Perera *et al.*, 1975). Dissecting microscopy, moreover, gives little indication of the pathological mechanism involved in producing villous abnormality. Histology must be used in any case for confirmatory purposes and would appear to provide a more rational basis for classification, but the dissecting microscope may still be useful for assessing the extent of structural villous abnormality.

Considerations of epithelial cell kinetics are also relevant to the

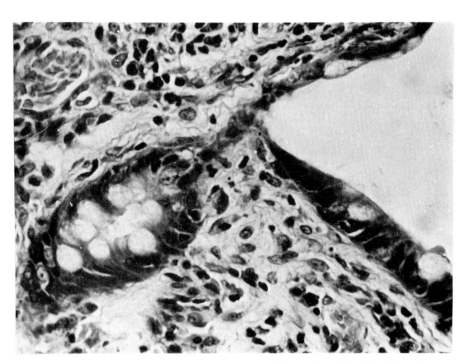

Fig. 4.14 Crypt abscess. Adhesions developing between epithelial cells at the crypt neck at a later phase of crypt abscess formation. HE × 525.

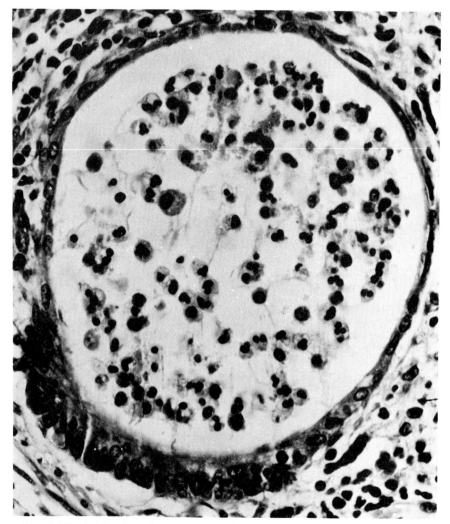

Fig. 4.15 Fully developed crypt abscess showing pronounced crypt distension. From a case of Crohn's disease. HE × 260.

classification of mucosal abnormalities. Shiner and Doniach (1960) noted that there was a close kinetic similarity between the epithelial cells of the small intestine and the haemopoietic system. Creamer (1965) took this a stage further and suggested that abnormal villous patterns might be analogous to haemolytic, hypoplastic or dyshaemopoietic forms of anaemia. Booth (1968) has pursued the haematological analogy to the cytological level and has described microcytic, normocytic and macrocytic types of epithelial disturbance in disease states. Although verification by radio-isotopic studies is lacking as yet, there is considerable indirect evidence to support these concepts.

The classification presented here takes these various factors into consideration, and is based primarily upon a simple histological evaluation of the dynamic state of the intestinal mucosa. It has been assumed that the haematological analogy is valid; in other words, that the relationship between the functional enterocyte population and the generative crypt epithelium is comparable to that existing between the peripheral blood cells and the haemopoietic cells of the bone marrow. This evaluation depends upon the measurement of three important variables: the villous height, which in broad terms is proportional to the enterocyte population; the crypt height, which provides an estimate of the extent of generative epithelial activity; and the ratio of crypt height to villous height, which is thought to be a function of enterocyte

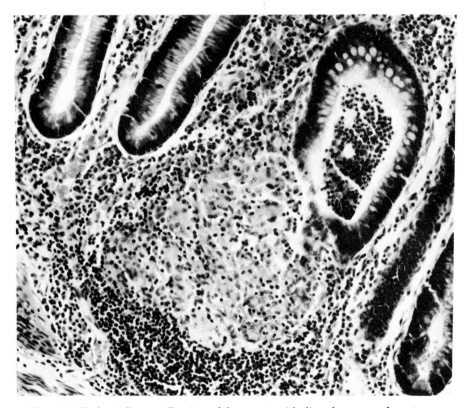

Fig. 4.16 Crohn's disease. Erosion of the crypt epithelium by a granulomatous lesion. HE × 210.

lifespan, While it is conceded that measurement of villous height does not take into account the extent to which finger villi are replaced by abnormal villous structures, it is undeniable that the severity of villous abnormality closely parallels the degree to which villous height is reduced. The technique used in measuring these variables has been described earlier (Section 2.5); it will be recalled that even in completely flat biopsies it may still be possible to measure these three variables if it is assumed that the upper limit of mitotic activity in the mucosa represents the dividing line between 'crypt' and 'villus' or, more precisely, 'surface' epithelium. The total mucosal height (Section 2.5) is also a useful measurement in 'flat' biopsies since a severe reduction may indicate a state of crypt-cell failure or hypoplasia (Section 4.2.3).

The normal villous pattern has been described in detail elsewhere (Section 3.2). In summary, the characteristic features are that the enterocyte population is appropriate to the locality in which the individual resides and that there is no reduction in the enterocyte lifespan. In the U.K. this means that the mean villous height should not be less than 300 microns (usually associated with a predominance of finger villi in the jejunum) and that the crypt: villus ratio should not exceed 0.6. In other localities a much lower villous height may be acceptable, although the crypt: villus ratio must be of the same order (Section 3.6, Table 3.1). In the great majority of cases a subjective estimate of the three major variables is all that is necessary for routine diagnostic purposes; direct measurement is, however, useful in the occasional doubtful case, and is essential in research studies. From such studies it has become apparent that there are three main types of villous abnormality: the atrophic (crypt hyperplastic) pattern; the hypertrophic pattern; and the hypoplastic pattern. The main features of these are summarized in Table 4.1.

4.2.1   *The atrophic pattern* (Crypt hyperplastic villous atrophy)

This is by far the commonest type of villous abnormality. The main features of this pattern are an absolute reduction in mean villous height (VH) below the acceptable lower limit of normality, and increase in mean crypt height (CH),* and an increase in the crypt: villus ratio (CH:VH) above 0.6. In some instances the increase in CH is so great that despite a dramatic fall in the VH the total mucosal height (TH, equal to CH + VH) remains within the normal range; usually however

---

*This increase is only evident when the atrophic mucosa is compared with normal controls on a statistical basis. In only about 15 per cent of cases of the atrophic pattern is the CH absolutely increased.

Table 4.1 The abnormal villous patterns.

Histological features	Atrophic pattern (Crypt hyperplastic VA)	Hypoplastic pattern (Crypt hypoplastic VA)	Hypertrophic pattern (Localized)
Villous height	Decreased (< 300 μm)	Decreased (< 300 μm)	Increased (> 550 μm)
Crypt height	Normal or increased	Normal or decreased	Usually increased
CH:VH	Increased (> 0.6)	Normal	Normal or increased
Total mucosal height	Decreased or normal	Decreased	Increased
Villous epithelium	Enterocytes abnormal at villous extremity: intra-epithelial lymphocytes increased	Enterocytes usually normal: occasionally damaged or megalocytic	Sometimes normal: commonly damaged with neutrophil infiltration
Crypt epithelium	Enteroblasts normal Paneth cells may be decreased in number: argentaffin cells may be increased	Enteroblasts may be atypical or megalocytic	Enteroblasts sometimes normal: often damaged with crypt abscess formation or gastric metaplasia
Lamina propria	Plasma cells increased: subepithelial collagen formation in some cases	Sometimes normal: effects of causative factor, e.g. ischaemia or irradiation may be evident	Non-specific inflammatory response with fibrosis in some cases: neutrophil infiltration occasionally
Mechanism	Impaired enterocyte lifespan with compensatory enteroblast hyperplasia	Enteroblast damage with impaired enterocyte production	Uncertain: pre-ulcerative changes probably caused by inflammatory reaction in lamina propria

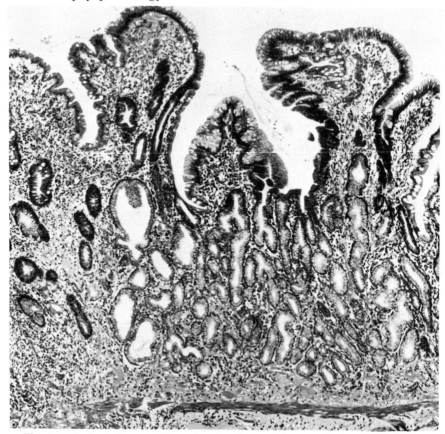

Fig. 4.17 Crohn's disease. There is extensive gastric metaplasia of pyloric type developing in relationship to the crypts of Lieberkuhn. HE × 72.

the TH is absolutely reduced. Within the enterocyte population it has been shown that there is an increase in the mitotic index (Section 3.5) which broadly parallels the increase in crypt height. As the VH falls, striking alterations in villous morphology take place. Initially the normal finger-villi are replaced by leaf-villi or short ridges (Fig. 4.37); with increasing VH reduction, long interdigitating ridges or convolutions develop; and ultimately the mucosal surface is reduced to a series of

Fig. 4.18 Crohn's disease. There is extensive gastric metaplasia of the villous epithelium. HE × 450.

Fig. 4.19 'Reflux' ileitis. Fully developed gastric metaplasia with clearly evident parietal cells in the ileal mucosa. Note that the metaplastic gastric tubules appear to be 'budding' from the villous epithelium. These changes arose as a consequence of ileo-rectal anastomosis for ulcerative colitis. HE × 450.

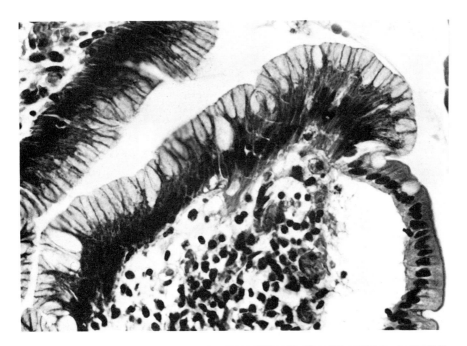
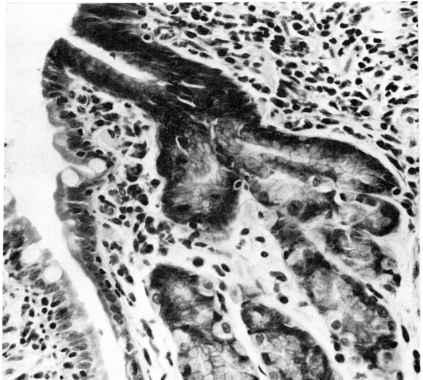

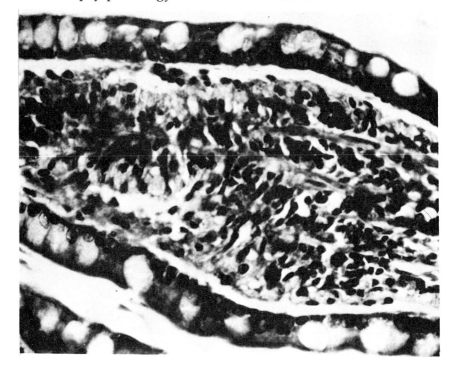

Fig. 4.20 Crohn's disease. Fibrosis developing in the lamina propria of a villus which also shows non-specific leucocytic infiltration. HE × 465.

mounds surrounded by a mosaic of troughs (Fig. 5.2), or becomes completely flat. In the 'convoluted' stage, where villus-like structures can still be detected histologically, the lesion has been described as partial villous atrophy (P.V.A., Fig. 4.38). In 'flat' biopsies, where discrete villi are no longer readily detectable, the condition is referred to as subtotal villous atrophy (S.V.A., Fig. 4.39). Functional enterocytes are not absent in S.V.A. since enzymatic studies have shown that some mature cells are invariably present in the upper part of the mucosa (Padykula *et al.*, 1961).

Other pathological phenomena accompany these villous changes. Of particular importance are changes in the enterocytes. The columnar cells at the villous extremity become distinctly abnormal, as revealed by a reduction in cell height, evidence of nuclear irregularity and loss of polarity, cytoplasmic basophilia or vacuolation, and, on occasion, syncytial change or tufting (Fig. 4.40). An increase in inflammatory cells, particularly plasma cells, is usual in the lamina propria, and there is an increase in intra-epithelial lymphocytes (Fig. 4.5).

(a) Pathogenesis In the majority of cases it would appear that the reduction in the enterocyte population observed in the atrophic pattern is due to accelerated loss of enterocytes from the villous surface, with compensatory hyperplasia of the regenerative crypt cells. The term villous atrophy is thus not entirely appropriate; in dynamic terms certainly few would regard haemolytic anaemia, which is a strictly comparable pathological process, as an 'atrophy' of the red cells. The term has however been hallowed by usage, at least in Britain. The hyperplasia of crypt cells accounts for the increase in crypt height and for the increased mitotic activity in the enterocyte population. The epithelial abnormalities at the villous extremity can be regarded as the morphological expression of premature enterocyte destruction, although from the study of early lesions it is apparent that the enterocytes emerging from the crypts are normal (Fig. 4.41). The effacement of the normal villous pattern and its replacement by ridges or convolutions, and ultimately by a flat structureless mucosa, is a further mani-

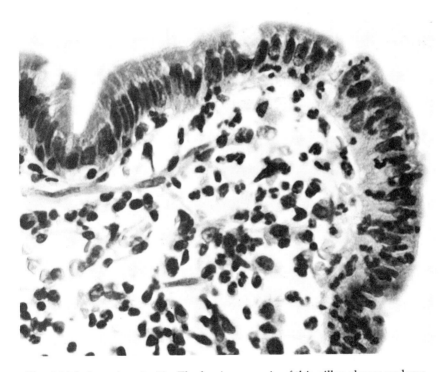

Fig. 4.21 Ischaemic enteritis. The lamina propria of this villus shows oedema, and neutrophils are emigrating from the blood vessels into the overlying villous epithelium. HE × 720.

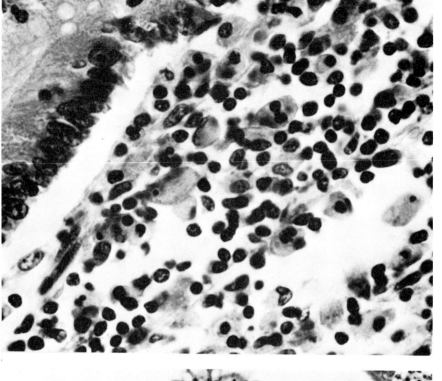
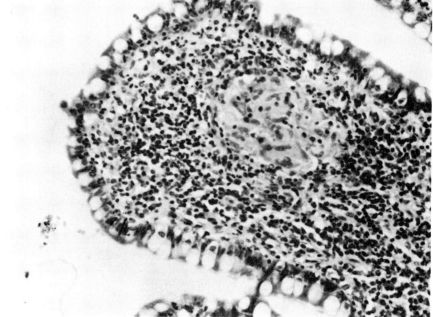

festation of a reduced enterocyte population, but the pathological mechanism underlying this process is not entirely clear. While villous fusion, possibly initiated by the formation of adhesions or 'synechiae' between abnormal epithelial cells, (Schenk *et al.*, 1967) may be a contributory factor, some observers hold the view that hypertrophy of intervillus ridges, produced by cells migrating from crypt orifices towards the villi, is responsible for the appearance of abnormal villous structures (Loehry and Creamer, 1969).

(b) *Clinical significance* The principal causes of villous atrophy as defined above are summarized in Table 4.2. It cannot be over-emphasized that coeliac disease accounts for the great majority of cases of subtotal villous atrophy in both children and adults in Britain and N. America, and even when this lesion is found in association with conditions such as dermatitis herpetiformis or hypogammaglobulinaemia or following gastric surgery, coeliac disease is often found to be responsible. The villous atrophy accompanying intestinal lymphoma is again often caused by pre-existing coeliac disease; this cannot always be established however, and when villous atrophy without obvious cause is found in an adult beyond middle age, the possibility that it is a manifestation of intestinal lymphoma merits serious consideration (Brunt *et al.*, 1969). Abnormal bacterial growth in the intestinal lumen, as seen in the 'stasis' or 'blind loop' syndrome, is capable of causing

Table 4.2 The main causes of the atrophic villous pattern.

Condition	Comment on mucosal lesions
Coeliac disease	Commonest cause of severe lesions in UK: due to gluten sensitivity
Stasis syndrome	Lesions limited to mucosa exposed to abnormal bacterial growth
Post-infective malabsorption	Transient lesions following intestinal infection in childhood
Tropical sprue	Usually mild lesions: possibly due to abnormal bacterial flora
Kwashiorkor	Severe lesions: reversed by improved nutrition

Fig. 4.22 Crohn's disease. A sarcoid follicle developing in the mucosal lamina propria. HE × 225.

Fig. 4.23 Typhoid fever. Histiocytes containing nuclear debris are prominent in the lamina propria of the ileum (autopsy case). HE × 820.

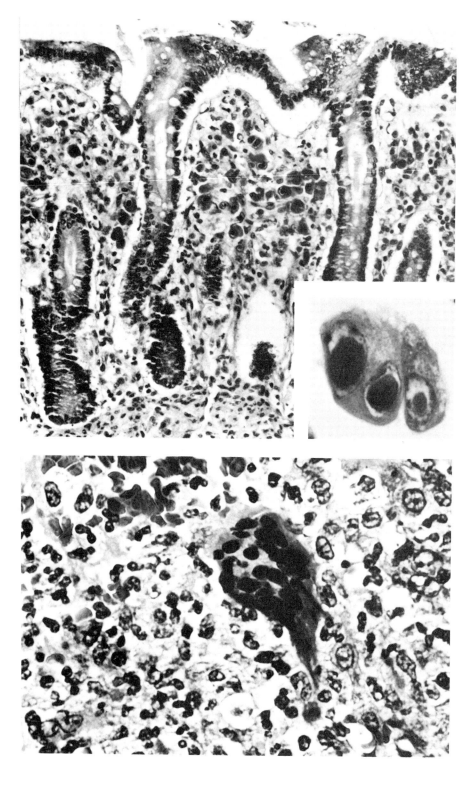

villous atrophy, usually of the partial type, although random jejunal biopsies in this condition rarely sample the affected area of the mucosa. Ultrastructural changes have been described in experimental blind loops (Gracey *et al.*, 1974). In childhood, transient villous atrophy is by no means uncommon following infective gastroenteritis (Section 7.5), and may on occasion be attributable to intolerance of cow's milk protein (Shiner *et al.*, 1975) or of soy protein (Ament and Rubin, 1972).

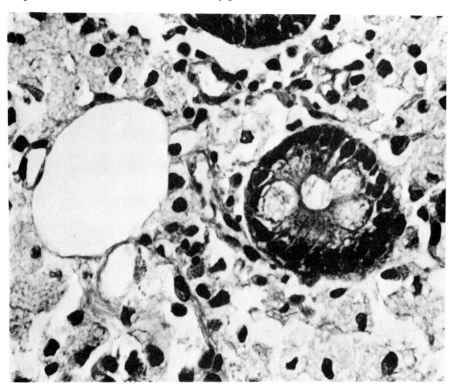

Fig. 4.26 Whipple's disease. The lamina propria contains numerous histiocytes the cytoplasm of which is stuffed with granules. Note also the 'clear space' without any clearly defined endothelial lining. HE × 720.

Fig. 4.24 Cytomegalic inclusion body disease. The mucosa of the small bowel is infiltrated by histiocytes containing the typical intranuclear inclusions. There is also a severe degree of villous atrophy. The patient was a child aged 18 months and had thymic hypoplasia (autopsy case). HE × 270. The insert (bottom right) shows the abnormal histiocytes in high power (× 720). Note the large intranuclear inclusions with surrounding zone clear of chromatin and in one cell a 'polar body'. The cytoplasm also contains inclusion bodies.
Fig. 4.25 Measles. Multinucleated Warthin-Finkeldey cells in the mucosa of a surgically removed appendix. HE × 720.

In the tropics, coeliac disease is rare, and the severe form of malnutrition known as kwashiorkor is a much more common cause of subtotal villous atrophy in childhood (Stanfield *et al.*, 1965). In adults S.V.A. is unusual; in some localities, tropical sprue is perhaps the commonest cause, although less severe forms of villous atrophy are more typical of this disease.

Minor or partial forms of villous atrophy have been reported in a large variety of disease states throughout the world (Table 4.3). Many of these reports have yet to be confirmed and should be regarded with caution (see Whitehead, 1971; Rubin and Dobbins, 1965; Roy-

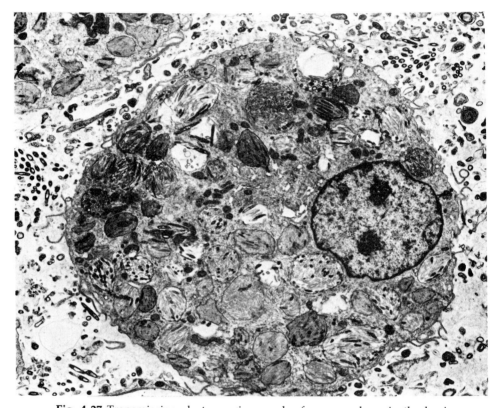

Fig. 4.27 Transmission electron micrograph of a macrophage in the lamina propria in a case of Whipple's disease. Around the macrophage can be seen numerous free rod-shaped organisms. Similar organisms are present within the macrophage, where they are gathered together in large numbers within the membrane-limited phagocytic vacuoles of the cell. The bacteria appear to be in different states of preservation, some being apparently still viable, while others are represented by apparently empty shells. These inclusions are responsible for the strong P.A.S. positivity of these macrophages. Micrograph by courtesy of Dr I. A. R. More.

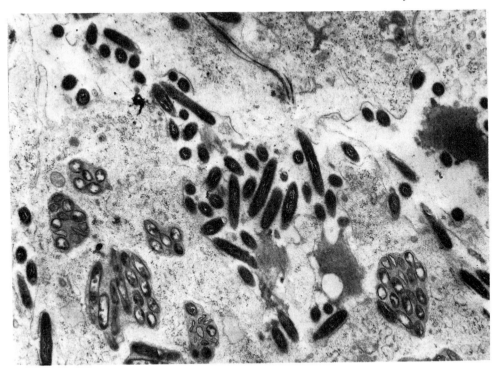

Fig. 4.28 Transmission electron micrograph of organisms in the lamina propria in a case of Whipple's disease. Details of the internal organization of the rod-shaped organisms can be made out in this micrograph. Several aggregates of partially disrupted organisms are seen within the macrophage cytoplasm.

Choudhury *et al.*, 1966); at least some have arisen from a failure to appreciate the extent of normal variation, especially in the tropical environment.

4.2.2 *The hypertrophic pattern*

This form of villous abnormality is not particularly well documented, since it is only rarely seen in random jejunal biopsies. It is, however, worthy of consideration as it is commonly found in surgical resections of small bowel, where it may give rise to diagnostic confusion. The main features of the pattern are absolute increases both in villous height (VH) and crypt height (CH), with the result that the total mucosal height is also greater than normal. There is no alteration in the CH:VH ratio or, presumably, in enterocyte lifespan, at least in the early stages.

The term villous hypertrophy is suitably applied to this condition, since the villi are increased in size without necessarily being increased

Table 4.3 Other recorded causes of the atrophic villous pattern

Condition	Comment on mucosal lesions	References
Intestinal lymphoma	Observed in about 40% of tumours: may be due to pre-existing C.D., but often symptom-less	1, 2, 3
Hypogammaglobulinaemia	Lesions usually due to associated C.D. or giardiasis	4, 5
Gastric surgery	Jejunal biopsy usually normal; severe lesions usually due to co-existing coeliac disease, only rarely to high acid levels. Hypoplastic villous atrophy may be seen in malnourished patients	6, 7, 8, 9
Crohn's disease	PVA usually: may be due to stasis	
Ulcerative colitis	Lesions usually mild: cause unknown	11, 12, 7
Giardiasis	Only in tropical cases or immunodeficient patients	13, 5
Ankylostomiasis	Probably not significant	14
Strongyloidiasis	Lesions unconvincing	15
Coccidiosis	Rare: may follow immuno-suppression	16, 17
Eosinophilic enteritis	Patchy lesions, more common in mucosal form of disease	18
Milk intolerance	Infants only: may be transient lesions; may be identical to C.D.	19
Soy-protein intolerance	Infants: lesions may be identical to C.D.	20
Dermatitis herpetiformis	Lesions due to associated C.D., but may be mild and variable	21, 22, 23
Acrodermatitis enteropathica	Lesions tend to be patchy: possibly due to zinc deficiency	24
Drug therapy	Neomycin, conovid: lesions of dubious significance	25, 26
Hepatic and pancreatic disease	Lesions described but unconvincing	27, 28, 29, 30
Zollinger–Ellison Syndrome	Patchy lesions of variable severity	31

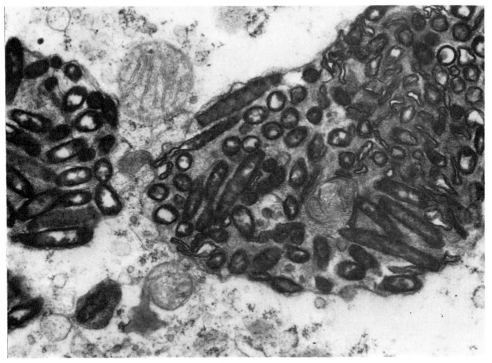

Fig. 4.29 Higher magnification view of rod-shaped organisms within phagocytic vacuoles of a Whipple's disease macrophage. The varying states of preservation of the organisms can be clearly seen. A limiting membrane surrounds the vacuole.

1. Lee (1966)
2. Gough, Read and Naish (1962)
3. Brunt, Sircus and McLean (1969)
4. Asquith (1974)
5. Ament and Rubin (1972a)
6. Scott, Williams and Clark (1964)
7. Roy-Choudhury et al. (1966)
8. Lee (1970)
9. Paulley, Fairweather and Leeming (1957)
10. Shiner and Drury (1963)
11. Salem, Truelove and Richards (1964)
12. Salem and Truelove (1965)
13. Wright, Tomkins and Ridley (1977)
14. Cook, Kajubi and Lee (1969)
15. Bras et al. (1964)
16. Trier et al. (1974)
17. Meisel et al. (1976)
18. Greenberger and Gryboski (1973)
19. Shiner et al. (1975)
20. Ament and Rubin (1972b)
21. Marks, Shuster and Watson (1966)
22. Scott et al. (1976)
23. Scott and Losowsky (1976)
24. Ament and Broviac (1973)
25. Jacobson, Chodos and Faloon (1960)
26. Watson and Murray (1966)
27. Astaldi and Strosselli (1960)
28. Hindle and Creamer (1965)
29. Conrad, Schwartz and Young (1964)
30. Rubin and Dobbins (1965)
31. Singleton, Kern and Waddell (1965)

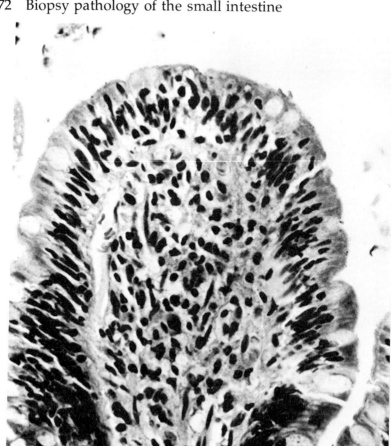

Fig. 4.30 Hypogammaglobulinaemia. There is marked reduction in plasma cells in the lamina propria. Note also the presence of *Giardia lamblia* in the lumen. HE × 500.

in number. Sometimes this is a diffuse change; it has been observed in experimental animals during lactation (Elias and Dowling, 1976) and following elemental nutrition (Nelson *et al.*, 1977), in both of which conditions there is probably a true enterocyte hyperplasia in response to functional demand. In man, enterocyte hyperplasia may occur as a compensatory phenomenon following massive intestinal resection (Porus, 1965). More often, however, it is pathological and localized, usually being found in the vicinity of gross ulcerative or stenotic lesions. In contrast to the diffuse 'physiological' or compensatory forms of villous hypertrophy referred to above, the villi in the pathological form are grossly thickened as a result of dense leucocytic infiltration, with a predominance of plasma cells. Congestion, oedema and eventually fibrosis of the lamina propria may be seen (Fig. 4.42). The villi, moreover, often show distortion in shape as a result of marked fibrous thickening towards the villous base, and pronounced attenuation of the villous extremity (Fig. 4.43).

Pathological villous hypertrophy can thus be seen as a manifestation of chronic mucosal inflammation which may vary greatly in intensity. As the inflammatory reaction becomes more severe, however, additional mucosal changes take place. Most striking is ablation of the normal villous architecture and its replacement by a flat mucosa,

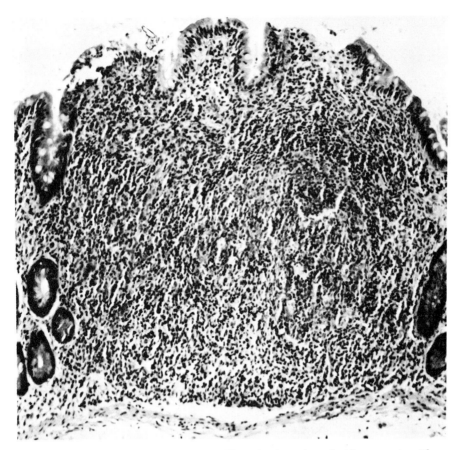

Fig. 4.31 Hypogammaglobulinaemia. There is a large lymphoid aggregate with prominent germinal centre formation ('nodular lymphoid hyperplasia'). HE × 180.

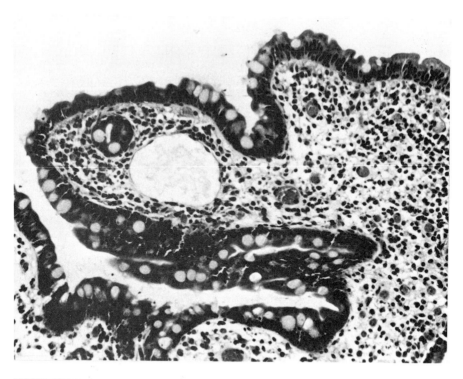
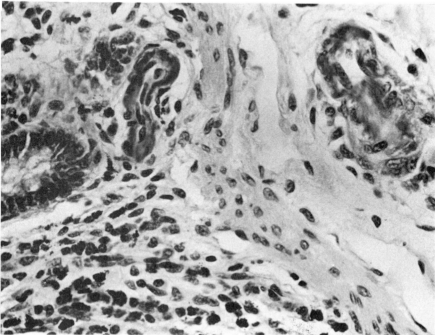

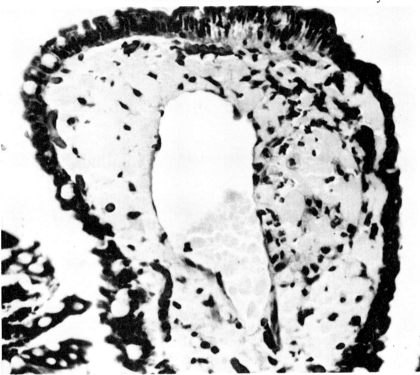

Fig. 4.34 Waldenströms macroglobulinaemia. The villous lamina propria is grossly distended by amorphous hyaline material giving a positive reaction with periodic-acid Schiff. The lacteals are also dilated and contain inspissated material and occasional foamy hisiocytes are seen in the lamina propria. HE × 330. Case kindly supplied by Dr D. C. Carfrae.

possibly as a result of villous fusion. This appearance could be described as 'pseudo-atrophy' since, while resembling subtotal villous atrophy, the total mucosal height is far in excess of the normal range (Fig. 4.44). Pseudo-atrophy is to be regarded as a sign of incipient mucosal breakdown. It is often associated with crypt abscess formation, which is also a pre-ulcerative lesion (Fig. 4.15), and with metaplastic change of pyloric type, which is a manifestation of recurrent epithelial damage (Fig. 4.17).

Fig. 4.32 Crohn's disease. Jejunal biopsy showing dilatation of the mucosal lymphatics. There is also an increase in small lymphocytes in the lamina propria. HE × 180.

Fig. 4.33 Amyloidosis. The blood vessels both in the mucosa and submucosa show amyloid deposition. HE × 450.

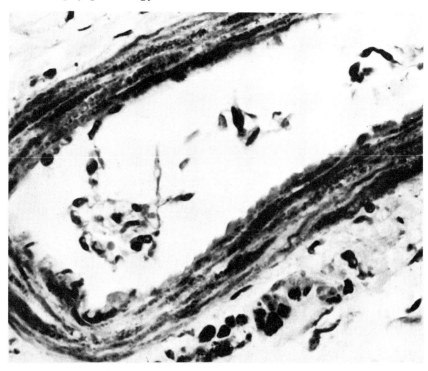

Fig. 4.35 Coeliac disease. The smooth muscle in a submucosal blood vessel shows marked lipofuscin deposition (autopsy case). HE × 635.

Occasionally, the hypertrophic state is observed undergoing transition to a true atrophic pattern (Section 4.2.1). This appears to arise through shedding of the often tenuous superficial portions of hypertrophic villi (Fig. 4.43). The residual villi are shortened or truncated, while the crypt height remains normal or increased; the CH:VH ratio thus rises, and the appearances become indistinguishable from P.V.A., although the vestiges of the shedding process may still be visible (Fig. 4.45). While this phenomenon is usually seen in localized villous lesions, a similar appearance has been observed in the 'blind loop' syndrome (Fig. 4.45) and tropical sprue (Fig. 5.5). It may be that the P.V.A. seen in these conditions has evolved from a hypertrophic pattern. Less often, true subtotal villous atrophy appears to arise from a hypertrophic mucosa; in this context S.V.A., like 'pseudo-atrophy' with which it is often associated, is a sign of incipient ulceration.

(a) Pathogenesis These villous changes are typically localized, and are always most prominent in the immediate vicinity of ulcerative and stenotic lesions. The causation of the pathological hypertrophic pat-

tern is uncertain. In all probability, however, an important factor is the abnormal bacterial proliferation which almost always complicates ulcerative or stenotic disease, regardless of its aetiology. It is also likely that the mucosa in the vicinity of such ulcerative or stenotic lesions is subjected to an exceptional degree of trauma, possibly resulting from fixation of the bowel wall and disturbed motility. In Crohn's disease, for example, Amman and Bockus (1961) have suggested that the mechanical stresses resulting from 'forced deformation' of the mucosal folds by submucosal oedema produces ulcerative lesions and enhances mucosal damage.

The hypertrophic pattern is not *primarily* an epithelial disturbance. The initial change is expansion of the lamina propria resulting from a non-specific chronic inflammatory reaction. The epithelial cells are thus called upon to provide an increased number of enterocytes to

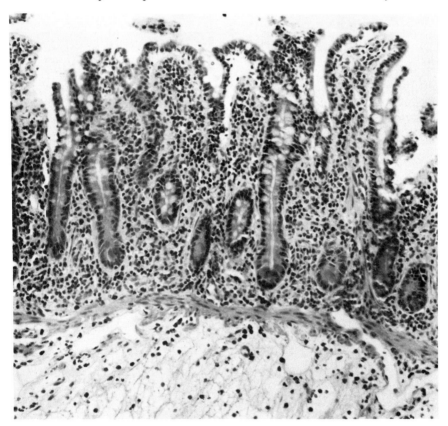

Fig. 4.36 Eosinophilic enteritis. There is pronounced submucosal oedema with eosinophil infiltration. The overlying mucosa shows partial villous atrophy. HE × 180.

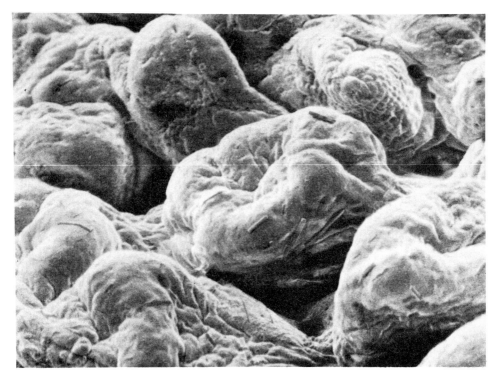

Fig. 4.37 Scanning electron micrograph of villous abnormalities in human duodenum. The short, squat, distorted villi seen here correspond to a picture of partial villous atrophy. Micrograph by courtesy of Dr K. E. Carr.

cover the expanded epithelial surface. In severe cases, however, the enterocytes themselves are damaged by the hostile environment and the adhesions forming between damaged enterocytes are probably responsible for the villous fusion which characterizes the state of 'pseudo-atrophy'. This lesion is always associated with ulceration and may be regarded as an attempt to 'cut back' the epithelial surface when its integrity is threatened. The appearance of true villous atrophy in similar circumstances is a further expression of increasing epithelial damage. It might be added that the crypt abscess (Fig. 4.17) observed particularly in colonic disease, but also found both in the small intes-

Fig. 4.38 Partial villous atrophy. Discrete villi are still visible, although markedly reduced in height. There is also a marked increase in the crypt:villus ratio. The patient suffered from intestinal lymphoma. HE × 180.

Fig. 4.39 Subtotal villous atrophy. Discrete villi are no longer visible and the mucosa appears completely flat. The crypts also appear to extend throughout the entire thickness of the mucosa. In this case the total mucosal height is greatly reduced (cf. Fig. 5.1). The patient suffered from intestinal lymphoma. HE × 180.

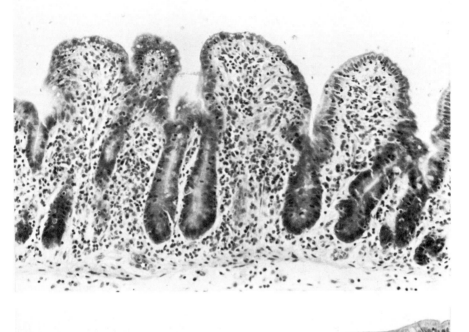

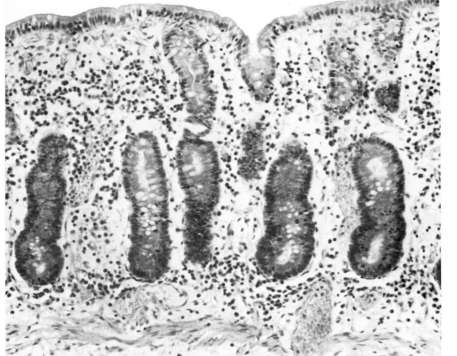

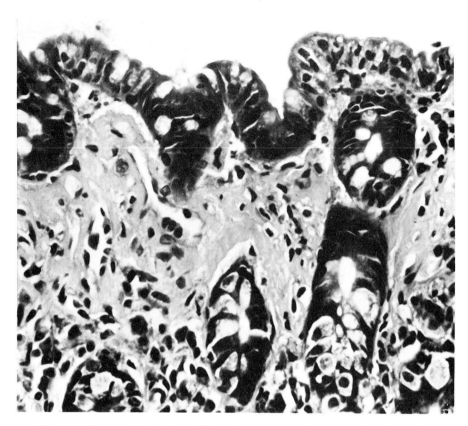

Fig. 4.40 The atrophic pattern. The enterocytes on the mucosal surface show reduction in height, vacuolation of the cytoplasm and nuclear irregularity. There is also pronounced sub-epithelial collagen formation ('collagenous sprue'). The patient suffered from coeliac disease. HE × 525.

tine and stomach – is a similar non-specific 'marker' of incipient breakage in epithelial continuity: it is produced by the emigration of neutrophils through micro-ulcers in the crypt epithelium; the subsequent crypt distension is due to the formation of occlusive adhesions at the crypt neck (Fig. 4.14).

(b) Clinical significance The hypertrophic pattern is entirely non-specific; while varying in severity, the same hypertrophic villous changes can be seen in association with such diverse conditions as Crohn's disease, tuberculosis, chronic peptic ulceration, malignant tumour or radiation enteritis. The same may be said of pathological phenomena such as crypt abscess formation and pyloric gland metaplasia, which commonly accompany those villous changes.

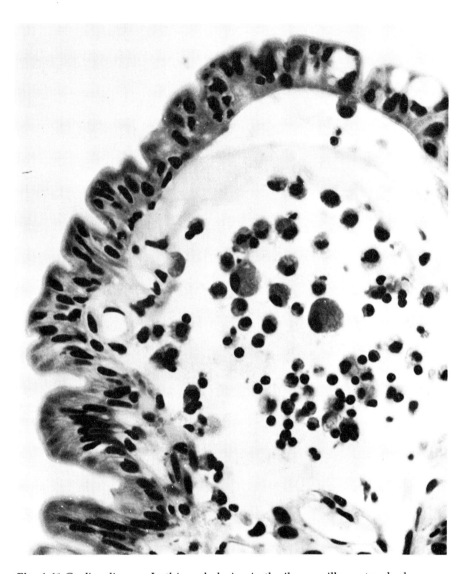

Fig. 4.41 Coeliac disease. In this early lesion in the ileum, villous atrophy has yet to develop, although the surface epithelium at the villous extremity is clearly abnormal. The enterocytes in the lower part of the villus, however, appear normal. Note also the prominent histiocytes in the oedematous lamina propria at the villous extremity. HE × 840.

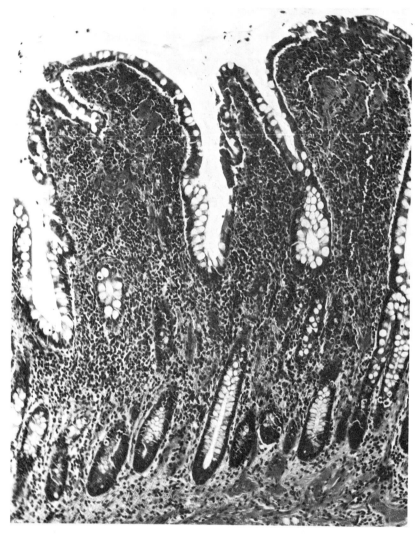

Fig. 4.42 Localized villous hypertrophy. The villi are increased in length and thickness, (the total mucosal height is 850 μm) and there is intense non-specific leucocytic infiltration with early collagen formation in the lamina propria. HE × 130.

4.2.3   *The hypoplastic pattern* (Crypt hypoplastic villous atrophy)

In this pathological pattern, an abnormally low villous height (VH) and a reduced crypt height (CH) produce a reduction of the total mucosal height, despite a normal CH:VH ratio. In certain biopsies which appear 'flat' histologically and would otherwise be classified as S.V.A.,

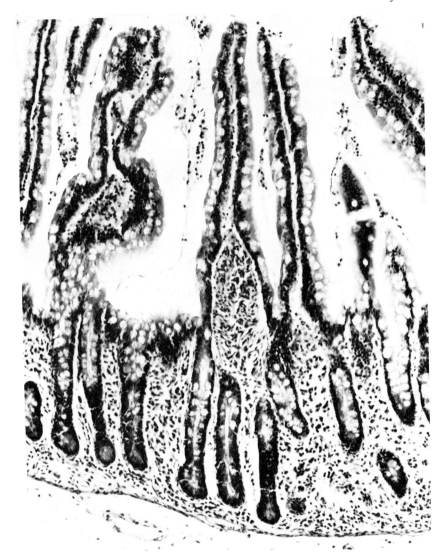

Fig. 4.43 Localized villous hypertrophy. The enlarged villi show pronounced attenuation of the villous extremity. HE × 180.

the total mucosal height is reduced to such an extent (usually less than 300 microns) as to suggest that crypt hyperplasia is absent, and that a hypoproliferative mechanism is involved (Fig. 4.46).

(a) *Pathogenesis* Presumably, there is a failure of the stem cells or enteroblasts to sustain a normal population of enterocytes, a condition

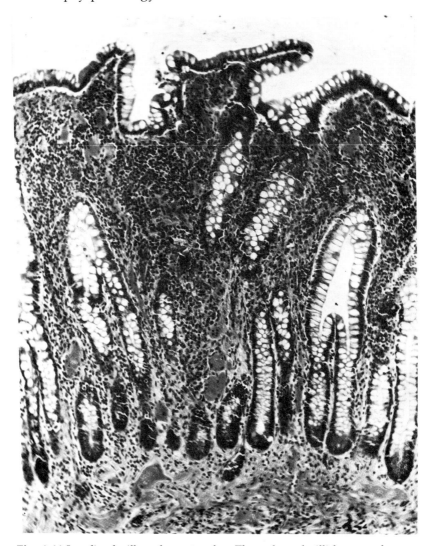

Fig. 4.44 Localized villous hypertrophy. The enlarged villi have undergone fusion to produce a 'flat' mucosal appearance ('pseudo-atrophy'). The total mucosal height is 850 μm. HE × 130.

corresponding to what Lipkin (1965) has described as 'hypoprolifera-tive cytopenia'. The maintenance of a normal CH:VH ratio, however, suggests that reduction in enterocyte lifespan is *not* of primary impor-tance in this pattern (cf. the atrophic pattern, Section 4.2.1). While the hypoplastic pattern is seldom found in intestinal biopsies, it seems probable that as the VH falls, changes in villous architecture similar to those found in the atrophic pattern (Section 4.2.1) take place, and hypoplastic variants of both P.V.A. and S.V.A. have been described.

In some instances there is cytological abnormality of the stem cells (Fig. 4.12) or irregularity of the crypts (Fig. 4.47) to support the view that interference with the normal process of cell replacement is either causing or contributing to the villous abnormality.

(b) Clinical significance Supposedly 'hypoplastic' forms of S.V.A. are rare. The best example is that observed in radiation enteritis, and some of the mucosal lesions resulting from ischaemia may also be of this nature. Similar changes have been seen following cytotoxic drug

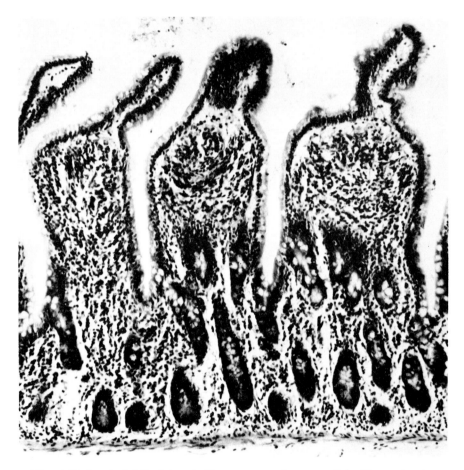

Fig. 4.45 Surgical 'blind loop'. The mucosa shows partial villous atrophy although the villi show attenuated processes at their extremities suggesting that the atrophic pattern may have evolved from a previously hypertrophic pattern. HE × 180.

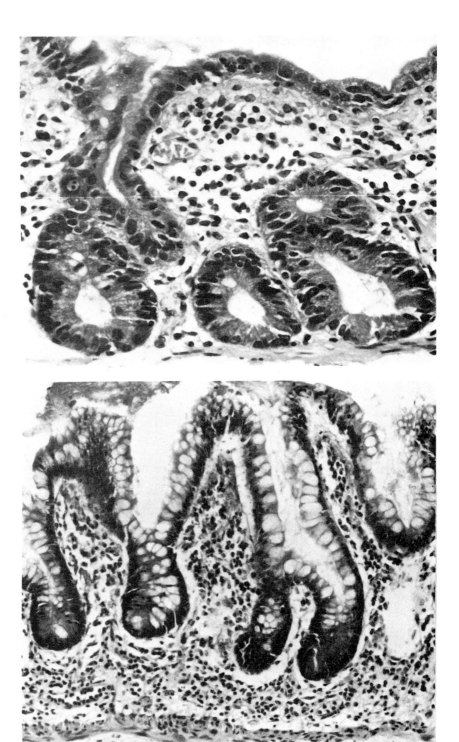

therapy in experimental animals (Clark and Harland, 1963): this is not however well documented in man. It is difficult if not impossible to detect minor forms of hypoplasia in the tropical environment, since the tropical normal pattern already appears to be distinctly hypoplastic by temperate standards. In the temperate environment, however, one occasionally encounters intestinal biopsies in which the VH is inappropriately reduced despite a normal CH:VH ratio ('hypoplastic P.V.A.' Fig. 4.48). This pattern is found mainly in patients who are either chronically ill or apparently undernourished (Creamer, 1965), e.g. following gastric surgery, and is presumably a morphological expression of reduced functional demand.

It is possible that in unusually severe cases of coeliac disease, in which the total mucosal height falls below 300 microns, a hypoplastic state may have supervened. This has been attributed to Paneth cell deficiency (Pink and Creamer, 1967) or irreversible stem cell damage. In some cases, cytomegalic changes have been observed in crypt cells, possibly as a result of complicating folic acid deficiency (Ten Thije, 1968) (see below). A similar marked depression of total mucosal height has also been found in some cases of tropical sprue (Swanson and Thomassen, 1965) and it is likely that the same mechanisms are implicated. In the severe state of infantile malnutrition, known as kwashiorkor, the predominant lesion is, however, true crypt hyperplastic S.V.A., (Stanfield et al., 1965) although severe states of hypoplasia have been found in fatal cases (Fig. 4.49).

There is still considerable doubt concerning the role of vitamin B12 deficiency and folic acid deficiency per se in the pathogenesis of structural villous abnormality. Moderate degrees of 'crypt hypoplastic villous atrophy' (Whitehead, 1971), cytomegalic changes in crypt cells, and macrocytic changes in enterocytes (Foroozan and Trier, 1967) have been described in vitamin B12 deficiency, but these are by no means constant and more controlled biopsy studies are required to confirm these findings. Similar hypoplastic changes have also been personally observed in some cases of folate deficiency (Figs. 5.14 and 5.15). In adults with this condition, however, the cytomegalic changes have

Fig. 4.46 The hypoplastic pattern. The mucosa appears completely 'flat' although the total mucosal height (185 μm) is reduced to such an extent as to suggest that a hypoproliferative mechanism is operating. Note that the epithelium both in the crypts and on the villous surface shows mild macrocytic change. This patient was thought on clinical grounds to be suffering from coeliac disease. HE × 450.

Fig. 4.47 The hypoplastic pattern. While villous structures are discernible they are markedly reduced in height, and the crypts are reduced in size and irregular in distribution. From a case of radiation enteritis. HE × 235.

been reported to be more patchy than in B12 deficiency (Hermos *et al.*, 1972) and in childhood cases crypt hyperplasia may be a feature (Davidson and Townley, 1977).

References

Amman, R. and Bockus, H. L. (1961), Pathogenesis of regional enteritis. *Archs. intern. Med.*, **107**, 504–513.

Ament, M. and Rubin, C. E. (1972a), Relation of giardiasis to abnormal intestinal structure and function in gastrointestinal immunodeficiency syndromes. *Gastroenterology*, **62**, 216–226.

Ament, M. and Rubin, C. E. (1972b), Soy protein – another cause of the flat intestinal lesion. *Gastroenterology*, **62**, 227–234.

Ament, M. and Broviac, J. (1973), Acrodermatitis enteropathica. Demonstration of small and large intestinal mucosal lesions: failure of hyperalimentation, intralipid and Diodoquin to reverse the intestinal lesions and generalized malabsorption syndrome. *Gastroenterology*, **64**, 692. (Abstract)

Ament, M. and Ochs, H. (1973), Gastrointestinal manifestations of chronic granulomatous disease. *New Engl. J. Med.*, **288**, 382–387.

Asquith, P. (1974), Immunology. In *Clinics on Gastroenterology 3, No. 1 (Coeliac disease)*, p. 213. Saunders, London.

Astaldi, G., Meardi, G. and Lisino, T. (1966), The iron content of jejunal mucosa obtained by Crosby's biopsy in haemochromatosis and haemosiderosis. *Blood*, **28**, 70–82.

Astaldi, G. and Strosselli, E. (1966), Peroral biopsy of the small intestine in hepatic cirrhosis. *Am. J. dig. Dis.*, **5**, 603–612.

Bras, G., Richards, R.C., Irvine, R. A., Milner, F. P. A. and Ragbeer, M. M. S. (1964), Infection with *Strongyloides stercoralis* in Jamaica. *Lancet*, **2**, 1257–1260.

Booth, C. C., Stewart, J. S., Holmes, R. and Brackenbury, W. (1962) Dissecting microscope appearance of intestinal mucosa. In *Ciba Foundation Study Group No. 14: Intestinal Biopsy*, (ed. Wolstenholme, G. E. W. and Cameron, M. P.), pp. 2–23. Churchill, London.

Booth, C. C. (1968), Enteropoiesis: Structural and functional relationships of the enterocyte. *Post-grad. med. J.*, **44**, 12–16.

Brunser, O., Castillo, C. and Araya, M. (1976), Fine structure of the small intestinal mucosa in infantile marasmic malnutrition. *Gastroenterology*, **70**, 495–507.

Brunt, P. W., Sircus, W. and McLean, N. (1969), Neoplasia and the coeliac syndrome in adults. *Lancet*, **1**, 180–184.

Cappell, D. F., Hutchison, H. E. and Jowett, M. (1957), Transfusional siderosis: the effects of excessive iron deposits on the tissues. *J. Path. Bact.*, **74**, 245–264.

Fig. 4.48 The hypoplastic pattern. The appearances resemble partial villous atrophy, although both the villi and the crypts are reduced in height. The patient suffered from malnutrition following gastric surgery. HE × 225.

Fig. 4.49 Kwashiorkor. The appearances of the jejunal mucosa in this autopsy case are markedly hypoplastic. HE × 180.

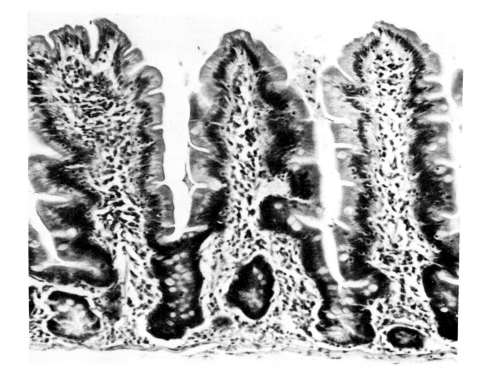

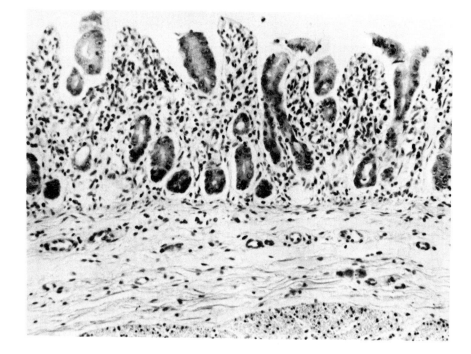

Clark, P. A. and Harland, W. A. (1963), Experimental malabsorption with jejunal atrophy induced by colchicine. *Br. J. exp. Path.*, **44**, 520–523.

Conrad, M. E., Schwartz, F. D. and Young, A. A. (1964), Infectious hepatitis – a generalized disease. *Am. J. Med.*, **37**, 789–801.

Cook, G. C., Kajubi, S. and Lee, F. D. (1969), Jejunal morphology of the African in Uganda. *J. Path.*, **98**, 157–169.

Creamer, B. (1965), The dynamics of the small intestinal mucosa. In *Recent Advances in Gastroenterology*. (Ed. Badenoch, J. and Brooke, B. N.), pp. 148–161. Little, Brown & Co., Boston.

Davidson, G. P. and Townley, R. R. W. (1977), Structural and functional abnormalities of the small intestine due to intestinal folic acid deficiency in infancy. *J. Pediat.*, **90**, 590–594.

Duque, E., Lotero, H., Boanos, O. and Mayoral, L. G. (1975), Enteropathy in adult protein malnutrition: ultrastructural findings. *Am. J. clin. Nutr.*, **28**, 914–924.

Elias, E. and Dowling, R. H. (1976), The mechanism for small bowel adaptation in lactating rats. *Clin. Sci. mol. Med.*, **51**, 427–433.

Erlandsen, S. L. and Chase, D. G. (1974), Morphological alterations in the microvillous border of villous epithelial cells produced by intestinal microorganisms. *Am. J. clin. Nutr.*, **27** 1277–1286.

Foroozan, P. and Trier, J. (1967), Mucosa of the small intestine in pernicious anaemia. *New Engl. J. Med.*, **277**, 553–559.

Gough, K. R., Read, A. E. and Naish, J. M. (1962), Intestinal reticulosis as a complication of idiopathic steatorrhoea. *Gut*, **3**, 232–239.

Gracey, M., Papadimitriou, J. and Bower, G. (1974), Ultrastructural changes in the small intestines of rats with self-filling blind loops. *Gastroenterology*, **67**, 646–651.

Greenberger, N. and Gryboski, J. D. (1973), In *Gastrointestinal Disease* (Ed. Sleisenger, M. H. and Fordtran, J. S.) pp. 1066–1082. Saunders, Philadelphia.

Hermos, J. A., Adams, W. H., Lio, Yong, K., Sullivan, L. W. and Trier, J. S. (1972), Mucosa of the small intestine in folate deficient alcoholics. *Ann. intern. Med.*, **76**, 957–965.

Hindle, W. and Creamer, B. (1965), Significance of a flat small intestinal mucosa. *Br. med. J.*, **2**, 455–459.

Hourihane, D.O'B. (1966), The pathology of malabsorptive states. In *Recent Advances in Pathology*, (Ed. Harrison, C. V.) 8th Ed. Churchill, London.

Jacobson, E. D., Priot, J. T. and Faloon, W. W. (1960), Malabsorptive syndrome induced by neomycin: morphologic alterations in the jejunal mucosa. *J. Lab. clin. Med.*, **56**, 245–250.

James, A. H. (1964), Gastric epithelium in the duodenum. *Gut*, **5**, 285–294.

Klima, M., Gyorkey, P., Min, K. W. and Gyorkey, F. (1977), Electron microscopy in the diagnosis of giardiasis. *Archs. Path.*, **101**, 133–135.

Lee, F. D. (1964), Pyloric metaplasia in the small intestine. *J. Path. Bact.*, **87**, 267–277.

Lee, F. D. (1970), *The intestinal mucosa in health and disease*. M.D. thesis, University of Dundee.

Lee, F. D., El-Ghobarey, A. F., Buchanan, W. W. and Browne, M. K. (1978), Rheumatoid arthritis, amyloidosis, intestinal ulceration, refractory iron deficiency anaemia and intestinal haemosiderosis: a new clinical syndrome? *Revue int. Rheumatol.*, **7**, 121–124.

Lewin, K. J., Harell, G. S., Lee, A. S. and Crowley, L. G. (1974), Malacoplakia. An electron microscopic study: demonstration of bacilliform organisms in malacoplakic macrophages. *Gastroenterology*, **66**, 28–45.

Liber, A. F. (1951), Aberrant pyloric glands in regional ileitis. *Archs. Path.*, **51**, 205–212.

Lipkin, M. (1965), Cell replication in the gastrointestinal tract of man. *Gastroenterology*, **48**, 616–624.

Loehry, C. A. and Creamer, B. (1969), Three-dimensional structure of the human small intestinal mucosa in health and disease. *Gut*, **10**, 6–12.

Maizel, H., Ruffin, J. M., and Dobbins, W. O., (1970), Whipple's disease: a review of 19 patients from one hospital and a review of the literature since 1950. *Medicine (Baltimore)*, **49**, 175–205.

Marks, J., Shuster, S. and Watson, A. J. (1966), Small bowel changes in dermatitis herpetiformis. *Lancet*, **2**, 1280–1282.

Meisel, J. L., Perera, D. R., Meligro, C. and Rubin, C. E. (1976), Overwhelming watery diarrhea associated with a cryptosporidium in an immunosuppressed patient. *Gastroenterology*, **70**, 1156–1160.

Merrill, T. G. and Sprinz, H. (1968), The effect of staphylococcal enterotoxin on the fine structure of the monkey jejunum. *Lab. Invest.*, **18**, 114–123.

Morningstar, W. A. (1975), Whipple's disease. An example of the value of the electron microscope in diagnosis, follow-up, and correlation of a pathologic process. *Human Pathol.*, **6**, 443–454.

Nelson, L. M., Carmichael, H. A., Russell, R. I. and Lee, F. D. (1978), Small intestinal changes induced by an elemental diet (vivonex) in normal rats. *Clin. Sci. mol. Med.*, **55**, 509–511.

Norris, H. T. and Majno, G. (1968), On the role of the ileal epithelium in the pathogenesis of experimental cholera. *Am. J. Path.*, **53**, 263–280.

Padykula, H. A., Strauss, E. W., Ladman, A. J. and Gardner, F. H. (1961), A morphologic and histochemical analysis of the human jejunal epithelium in non-tropical sprue. *Gastroenterology*, **40**, 735–765.

Patrick, W. J., Denham, D. and Forrest, A. P. (1974), Mucous change in the human duodenum: a light and electron microscopic study and correlation with disease and gastric acid secretion. *Gut*, **15**, 767–776.

Paulley, J. W. (1954), Observations on the aetiology of idiopathic steatorrhoea. Jejunal and lymph node biopsies. *Br. med. J.*, **2**, 1318–1321.

Paulley, J. W., Fairweather, F. A. and Leeming, A. (1957), Post-gastrectomy steatorrhoea and patchy jejunal atrophy. *Lancet*, **1**, 406–407.

Perera, D., Weinstein, W. M. and Rubin, C. E. (1975), Small intestinal biopsy. *Human Path.*, **6**, 157–217.

Pink, I. J. and Creamer, B. (1967), Response to a gluten free diet of patients with coeliac syndrome. *Lancet*, **1**, 300–304.

Porus, R. L. (1956), Epithelial hyperplasia following massive small bowel resection in man. *Gastroenterology*, **48**, 753–757.

Pruzanski, W., Warren, R., Goldie, J. and Katz, A. (1973), Malabsorption syndrome with infiltration of the intestinal wall by extracellular monoclonal macroglobulin. *Am. J. Med.*, **54**, 811–818.

Ranchod, M. and Kahn, L. B. (1972), Malacoplakia of the gastrointestinal tract. *Archs. Path.*, **94**, 90–97.

Roy-Choudhury, D., Cooke, W. T., Tan, D. T., Banwell, J. G. and Smits, B. J. (1966), Jejunal biopsy: criteria and significance. *Scand. J. Gastroenterol.*, **1**, 57–74.

Rubin, C. E., Brandborg, L. L., Phelps, P. C. and Taylor, H. C. (1960), Studies in coeliac disease. I. The apparent identical and specific nature of the duodenal and proximal jejunal lesion in coeliac disease and idiopathic sprue. *Gastroenterology*, **38**, 28–49.

Rubin, C. E., Brandborg, L. L., Flick, A. L., Phelps, P. C., Parmentier, C. and van Neil, S. (1962), Studies in coeliac sprue. III. The effect of repeated wheat instillation into the proximal ileum in patients on a gluten free diet. *Gastroenterology*, **43**, 621–641.

Rubin, C. E. and Dobbins, W. O. (1965), Peroral biopsy of the small intestine. A review of its diagnostic usefulness. *Gastroenterology*, **49**, 676–697.

Rubin, E., Rybak, B. J., Lindenbaum, J., Gerson, C. D., Walker, G. and Lieber, C. S. (1972), Ultrastructural changes in the small intestine induced by ethanol. *Gastroenterology*, **63**, 801–814.

Salem, S. N., Truelove, S. C. and Richards, W. C. D. (1964), Small intestinal and gastric changes in ulcerative colitis: a biopsy study. *Br. med. J.*, **1**, 394–398.

Salem, S. N. and Truelove, S. C. (1965), Small intestinal and gastric abnormalities in ulcerative colitis. *Br. med. J.*, **1**, 827–831.

Sanusi, I. D. and Tio, F. O. (1974), Gastrointestinal malacoplakia. Report of a case and a review of the literature. *Am. J. Gastroent.*, **62**, 356–366.

Schenk, E. A., Samloff, I. M. and Klipstein, F. A. (1967), Pathogenesis of jejunal mucosal alterations: synechia formation. *Am. J. Path.*, **50**, 523–528.

Scott, B. B., Young, S., Rajah, S. M., Marks, J. and Losowsky, M. S. (1976), Coeliac disease and dermatitis herpetiformis: further studies of their relationship. *Gut*, **17**, 759–762.

Scott, B. B. and Losowsky, M. S. (1976), Patchiness and duodenal-jejunal variation of the mucosal abnormality in coeliac disease and dermatitis herpetiformis. *Gut*, **17**, 984–992.

Scott, G. B., Williams, M. J. and Clark, C. G. (1964), Comparison of jejunal mucosa in post-gastrectomy states, idiopathic steatorrhea and controls using the dissecting microscope and conventional histological methods. *Gut*, **5**, 553–562.

Sheehy, T. M., Artenstein, M. S. and Green, R. W. (1964), Small intestinal mucosa in certain viral diseases. *J. Am. med. Ass.*, **190**, 1023–1028.

Shiner, M. and Doniach, I. (1960), Histopathologic studies in steatorrhoea. *Gastroenterology*, **38**, 419–440.

Shiner, M. and Drury, R. A. B. (1962), Abnormalities of the small intestinal mucosa in Crohn's disease (regional enteritis). *Am. J. dig. Dis.*, **7**, 744–759.

Shiner, M., Ballard, J., Brook, C. G. D., Herman, S. and Lovell, D. (1975), Jejunal biopsy in the management of infants suspected of cow's milk protein intolerance. *Gut*, **16**, 822 (Abstract).

Singleton, J. W., Kern, F. and Waddell, W. R. (1965), Diarrhea and pancreatic islet cell tumour. Report of a case with severe jejunal mucosal lesion. *Gastroenterology*, **49**, 197–208.

Stanfield, J. P., Hutt, M. S. R. and Tunnicliffe, R. (1956), Intestinal biopsy in kwashiorkor. *Lancet*, **2**, 519–523

Stewart, J. S., Pollock, D. J., Hoffbrand, A. V., Mollin, D. L. and Booth, C. C. (1967), A study of proximal and distal intestinal structure and absorptive function in idiopathic steatorrhoea. *Q. J. Med.*, **36**, 425–444.

Swanson, V. L. and Thomassen, D. V. M. (1965), Pathology of the jejunal mucosa in tropical sprue. *Am. J. Path.*, **46**, 511–551.

Ten Thije, O. (1963), Darmslijmvkes en Spruw (Intestinal mucosa and sprue). Doctoral thesis, University of Groningen, July 1963, 179 pp.

Trier, J. S., Moxey, P. C., Schimmel, E. M. and Robles, E. (1974), Chronic intestinal coccidiosis in man: intestinal morphology and response to treatment. *Gastroenterology*, **66**, 923–935.

Trier, J. S., Phelps, P. C., Eidelman, S. and Rubin, C. E. (1965), Whipple's disease: light and electron microscope correleation of jejunal mucosal histology with antibiotic treatment and clinical status. *Gastroenterology*, **48**, 684–707.

Trowell, H. C., Davies, J. N. P. and Dean, R. F. A. (1954). In *Kwashiorkor*, pp. 149–150. Edward Arnold, London.

Ward, M., Eastwood, M. A. and Ferguson, A. (1976), Jejunal lysozyme and Paneth cell population in coeliac disease. *Gut*, **17**, 813 (Abstract).

Watson, A. J. and Roy, A. D. (1960), Paneth cells in the large intestine in ulcerative colitis. *J. Path. Bact.*, **80**, 309–316.

Watson, W. C. and Murray, D. (1966), Lactase deficiency and jejunal atrophy associated with administration of conovid. *Lancet*, **1**, 65–67.

Whitehead, R. (1971), The interpretation and significance of morphological abnormalities in jejunal biopsies. In *Intestinal Absorption and its Derangements*, (Ed. Dawson, A. M.), *J. Clin. Path.*, **24**, Suppl. (Roy. Coll. Path.) **5**, 108–124.

Wright, R. G., Tomkins, A. M. and Ridley, D. S. (1977), Giardiasis: clinical and therapeutic aspects. *Gut*, **18**, 343–350.

Yokoyama, I., Kozuka, S., Ito, K., Kubota, K., Yokoyama, Y. and Kondo, T. (1977), Gastric gland metaplasia in the small and large intestine. *Gut*, **18**, 214–218.

Part Two: Mucosal disease

As mentioned previously, *in vivo* biopsy techniques are particularly effective in the diagnosis of disease processes which produce diffuse lesions of the intestinal mucosa. Only rarely does random intestinal biopsy detect localized disease, which includes most neoplasms, or patchy diseases, such as Crohn's disease. The only exception to this generalization is disease of the first part of the duodenum, which can be directly visualized by fiberscopic endoscopy, thus enabling focal lesions to be subjected to biopsy. For clinical purposes, therefore, the following discussion of mucosal disease has been placed under five headings; the causes of diffuse villous abnormality; malabsorptive states with distinctive pathological changes; mucosal abnormalities in other disease states; duodenitis; and tumours of the small intestine.

5 Diffuse villous abnormality

Following the widespread introduction of biopsy techniques villous abnormalities were reported in association with a large number of disease states. As the definition of villous abnormality has become more stringent, and the range of normal variation more fully appreciated, it has become apparent that there are relatively few causes of diffuse villous abnormality as defined in Section 4.2 (see Roy-Choudhury *et al.*, 1966). In the West of Scotland, for example, subtotal villous atrophy in adults is almost always caused by coeliac disease; other types of villous abnormality, such as the hypoplastic or hyperplastic states, are only rarely seen in biopsies. Thus, we will only discuss those conditions in which the presence of diffuse villous abnormality has been unequivocally established as the predominant intestinal lesion.

5.1 Coeliac disease

This condition, probably the most important cause of intestinal malabsorption in the developed world, is caused by a pathological response to the presence in the intestinal lumen of the dietary protein gluten, which is a constitutent of several cereals, especially wheat, rye, barley and oats. Clinical and pathological improvement following the exclusion of gluten from the diet is thus the all-important diagnostic feature. There is evidence suggesting that the abnormal response to gluten is genetically determined and closely related to inheritance of the histocompatibility antigen HLA-8 (Falchuk *et al.*, 1972). The mechanism whereby gluten, or a toxic fraction of gluten, exerts its effects on susceptible individuals is uncertain, although an immunological basis seems likely. In this context it is of interest that lesions similar to those of coeliac disease have been attributed to intolerance of cow's milk protein (Shiner *et al.*, 1975) or of soy protein (Ament and Rubin, 1972b). While the defect in coeliac disease, and its intestinal lesions, are in all probability present from infancy, the clinical effects are not always evident in childhood and may be delayed well into adult life. Most cases of the condition formerly known as idiopathic steatorrhoea are adult forms of coeliac disease. In less severe forms of the disease it seems likely that clinical disturbance is precipitated by unusually high gluten intake, intestinal infection or surgical procedures, especially those involving gastro-jejunal anastomosis.

Histological examination of a biopsy taken from the proximal jejunum or distal duodenum in untreated cases almost always shows subtotal villous atrophy of the 'crypt hyperplastic' type (Section 4.2.1 Fig. 5.1); and the dissecting microscope or scanning electron microscope correspondingly reveals a completely flat, or at best a mosaic, pattern, (Fig. 5.2). Marsh *et al*. (1970) and Marsh (1972) have documented these features in detail. The intestinal crypts open into common vestibules which are surrounded by a heaped-up collar of enterocytes. Between these raised collars, the cobblestone patterns of individual enterocytes can be seen. With dietary exclusion a progressive regrowth of the villous pattern can be traced through the stages of ridge and convolution formation.

As might be expected, the mucosal lesions of coeliac disease are always most severe in the proximal parts of the small bowel although not necessarily more severe in the distal duodenum than in the proximal jejunum; more distally the mucosa undergoes transition to partial villous atrophy and may become virtually normal in the terminal parts of the ileum. The mildest lesions of coeliac disease are thus best appreciated in these distal sites (Fig. 5.3). As a corollary, the proximal parts of the small bowel are the last to show improvement following the removal of gluten from the diet; indeed the upper jejunum may never revert entirely to normal, except perhaps in childhood (see Fig. 5.2).

In a small proportion of untreated cases, jejunal biopsy reveals partial, as opposed to subtotal, villous atrophy (Fig. 5.3). This is particularly common in the form of coeliac disease associated with dermatitis herpetiformis (Section 5.3) and may indicate a relatively mild expression of gluten intolerance. Less easy to understand are those rare

---

Fig. 5.1(a) Coeliac disease. Subtotal villous atrophy, the typical appearance of the jejunal mucosa in an untreated case. HE × 180.
(b) Scanning electron micrograph of mucosal surface in coeliac disease. There is a complete absence of villi. The crypt mouths are surrounded by raised mounds of cells, forming collars around their orifices. The cell outlines are relatively prominent, as is common in coeliac disease. Micrograph by courtesy of Dr K. E. Carr.

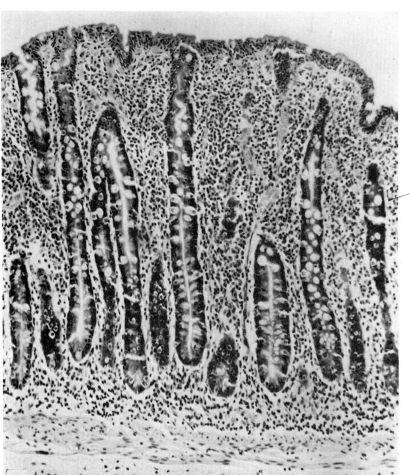

Sub. total
villous
atrophy.

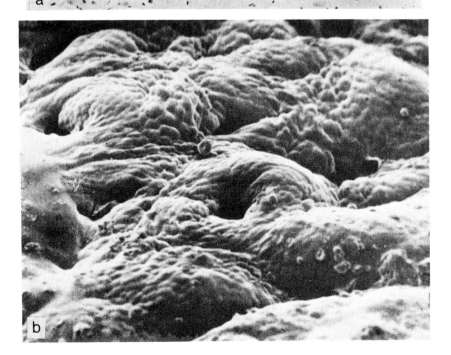

mild partial

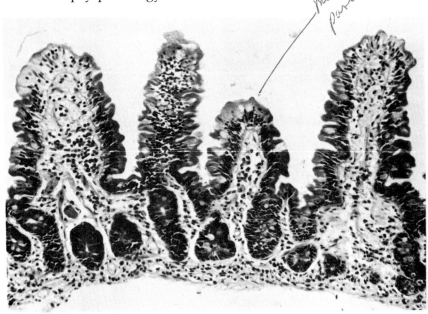

Fig. 5.2 Coeliac disease. In this treated case mild partial villous atrophy persists, and the enterocytes at the villous extremity still show mild abnormality. HE × 180.

cases of coeliac disease in which the initial jejunal biopsy appears to be normal (Challacombe *et al.*, 1975). It is notable, however, that in surgically resected portions of small bowel affected by coeliac disease the mucosal lesions are always maximal at the tips of mucosal folds, and may be minimal or absent in the troughs between folds. There is thus a possibility that the biopsy capsule might sample the unrepresentative but relatively normal mucosa in the latter sites. On grounds of probability, repeat biopsy should reveal the true state of the mucosa in such instances.

Some of the histological features of coeliac disease deserve special mention, although it has to be emphasized that none of these is specific. Of particular importance are the degenerative changes in the enterocytes or absorptive epithelial cells, which lose their tall columnar

Fig. 5.3(a) Coeliac disease. Severe partial villous atrophy of the jejunal mucosa in an untreated case. HE × 180.
(b) Coeliac disease. The atrophic mucosal pattern with the mucosal compartments outlined diagrammatically. Note that in comparison with Fig. 3.4b the villous compartment is greatly reduced, while the crypt compartment is markedly increased. HE × 180.

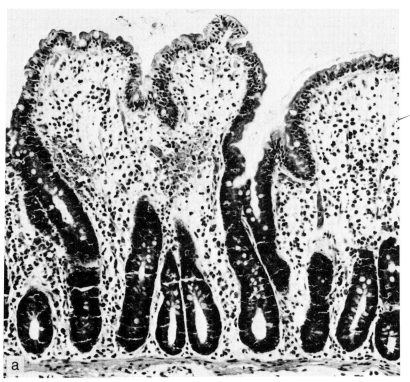

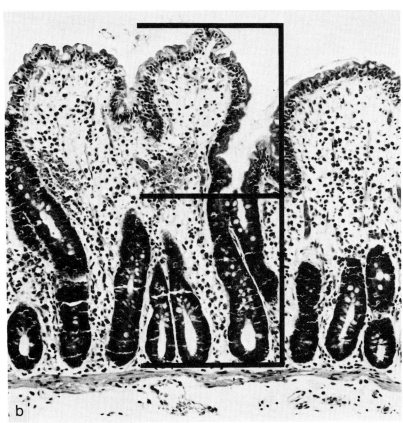

partial
villous
atrophy

shape and become markedly reduced in height. The cytoplasm becomes basophilic, and the nuclei irregular in shape and orientation (Fig. 4.5). Electron microscopy shows that the microvilli are stunted and irregular (Fig. 4.6). From the study of early lesions, however, it is apparent that the enterocytes emerging from the crypts appear normal and only exhibit degenerative changes as the villous extremity is approached (Fig. 4.41).

Of considerable interest is the marked increase in the number of intra-epithelial lymphocytes found in coeliac disease. Sometimes these lymphocytes equal or exceed the number of enterocytes (Ferguson and Murray, 1971), and give the impression of greatly increased cellularity in the surface epithelium (Fig. 4.5; see also Section 4.2.1). In contrast, lymphocytes are sparse in the lamina propria except in the vicinity of lymphoid aggregates. The increased cellularity of the lamina propria is due almost entirely to a pronounced increase in the number of plasma cells (Fig. 4.5). Eosinophils and histiocytes are, of course, present but are not apparently increased in number, although histiocytes are sometimes prominent in early lesions at the villous extremity (Fig. 4.41) and neutrophils can occasionally be demonstrated.

The markedly hyperplastic crypts, which might account for 90 per cent or more of the total mucosal height (Section 4.2.1), appear to include normal or slightly increased numbers of both goblet cells and intestinal endocrine cells. On the other hand, Paneth cells have been found to be reduced in number both before and after treatment (Ward *et al.*, 1976). In a small group of cases characterized by an unusually severe degree of villous atrophy, Paneth cells are virtually absent and there is a poor response to gluten withdrawal (Pink and Creamer, 1967). Although this state of 'Paneth cell deficiency' might be a specific disease entity, it probably represents a refractory variant of coeliac disease.

Another histological change occasionally associated with a severe degree of villous atrophy is the subepithelial formation of collagen (Fig. 4.40). A poor response to gluten withdrawal has also been observed in some patients with pronounced collagen deposition and the term 'collagenous sprue' has been applied to such cases, with the implication that they are distinct from coeliac disease (Weinstein *et al.*, 1970). Milder forms of collagen deposition can, however, be quite often demonstrated in subtotal villous atrophy responding to treatment in the usual way (Bossart *et al.*, 1975), and it seems probable that 'collagenous sprue' represents another potentially refractory form of coeliac disease.

Recurrent non-specific intestinal ulceration is a well recognized complication of coeliac disease, and the condition known as 'ulcerative jejunitis' is probably an expression of this phenomenon (Bayless *et al.*, 1967). While this complication cannot readily be detected by intestinal biopsy, there is evidence that it is especially associated with the state of 'collagenous sprue' referred to above (Jeffries *et al.*, 1968) or to the development of a state of crypt hypoplasia (Barry *et al.*, 1970). The detection of pyloric metaplasia in a biopsy might also raise the suspicion of an ulcerative process (Section 4.1.2). This change is particularly evident in cases of coeliac disease in which some form of gastro-jejunal anastomosis has been performed following peptic ulceration (Fig. 5.4; see also Section 5.6). Metaplastic change is not a feature of uncomplicated coeliac disease.

An interesting feature of some diagnostic value in coeliac disease is lipofuscin deposition in the intestinal smooth muscle (Fig. 4.35). This is particularly evident in autopsy cases, (Adlersberg and Schein, 1947) in

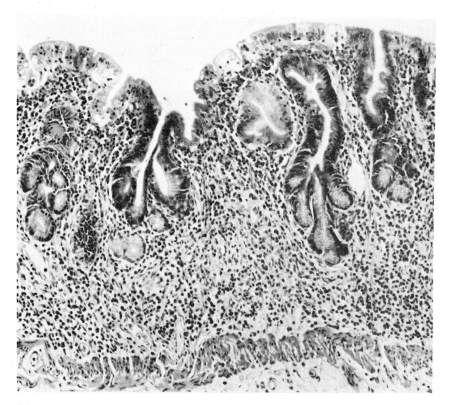

Fig. 5.4 Coeliac disease. There is subtotal villous atrophy, although the crypts are irregular and there is evidence of gastric metaplasia. The latter two changes were due to gastrojejunal anastomosis with recurrent stomal ulceration. HE × 180.

which the small intestine might have a distinctly brown colour macro-scopically. This change, which is probably a manifestation of either vitamin E deficiency (Mason and Telford, 1947) or protein-losing enteropathy (Schwartz and Jarnum, 1959) is not often seen in biopsies since it is most obvious in the smooth muscle of the muscularis propria close to Auerbach's plexus, and is only occasionally seen in the lamina muscularis mucosae.

Finally, mention must be made of the most serious complication of coeliac disease, which is the development of primary intestinal lym-phoma. While this tumour can seldom be detected by intestinal biopsy, it has been suggested that its onset can be predicted through the detection of certain deviations from the usual histological pattern observed in coeliac disease. The presence of an exceptionally dense leucocytic infiltrate in the lamina propria, especially when accom-panied by the presence of atypical lymphoid cells ('progressive hyper-plasia') (Whitehead, 1971) or an unusually high proportion of small lymphocytes in the infiltrate, (Ferguson et al., 1974) have been regarded as particularly significant in this respect. Intestinal lym-phoma has also been observed to arise in a case of 'collagenous sprue' (Jeffries et al., 1968; Whitehead, 1971). While the value of these obser-vations has yet to be fully established, they point to the possible diagnostic importance of detailed analysis of the biopsy appearances in coeliac disease (Section 9.3).

5.2 Tropical sprue

As the term implies, this malabsorptive disease is only encountered in certain geographical areas, particularly the Indian subcontinent, South-east Asia and Central America. It is thought to be uncommon in Africa, although this might be due in part to a failure of recognition (Thomas and Clain, 1976). The disease can affect those native to the tropics as well as visitors. While the cause remains unknown, abnor-mal bacterial growth in the intestinal lumen has been detected by the use of biopsy techniques, (Gorbach et al., 1969) and clinical improve-ment follows the administration of oral broad-spectrum antibiotics (Sheehy and Perez-Santiago, 1961). Indeed, in some respects the malabsorptive defect in tropical sprue resembles that of the blind loop syndrome, especially with regard to the frequency of vitamin B12 malabsorption (Banwell and Gorbach, 1969; Section 5.4). The improvement of the pathological changes in the intestinal mucosa following folic acid therapy (Sheehy et al., 1962) suggests however, that factors other than abnormal bacterial colonization may contribute to the pathogenesis of tropical sprue.

Jejunal biopsies in tropical sprue have been described as showing considerable variation in histological appearance (Brunser et al., 1970). At one end of the spectrum are biopsies which show such minor changes that it is difficult if not impossible to distinguish between them and biopsies from normal tropical residents (Section 3.2; see also Baker et al., 1962). On the other hand, frank subtotal villous atrophy has been observed in some cases (Swanson and Thomassen, 1965). In most instances, however, the changes are of an intermediate degree and correspond to partial villous atrophy (Butterworth and Perez-Santiago, 1958) characterized by a reduction in villous height associated with crypt hyperplasia, increased mitotic activity and abnormality of the villous epithelium (Fig. 5.5). The mucosal changes are therefore similar in pattern, if not in degree, to those of coeliac disease and only minor differences have been described. Thus eosinophils as well as plasma cells appear to be increased in number in the lamina propria, and a striking increase in argentaffin cells has been reported (Swanson and

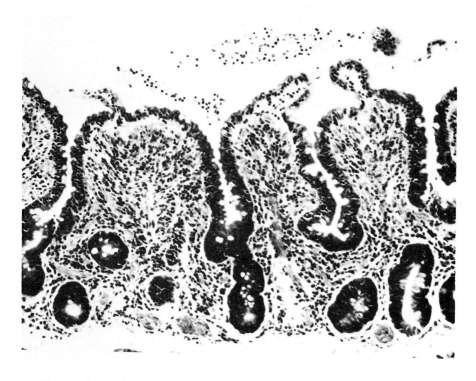

Fig. 5.5 Tropical sprue. The jejunal mucosa shows partial villous atrophy in this case. Note the slightly attenuated villous extremities, similar to the appearance sometimes observed in surgical blind-loops (Fig. 4.45). HE × 180.

Thomassen, 1965). One other interesting feature worthy of mention is that, in the most atrophic biopsies, crypt hyperplasia and mitotic activity tend, unexpectedly, to become less pronounced suggesting that the severity of the changes is due in such cases to the development of crypt hypoplasia (Swanson and Thomassen, 1965). It is tempting to attribute this to folic acid or vitamin B12 deficiency, which might help to explain the response of the mucosal lesions to folic acid administration. While the extent of the mucosal lesion in the small bowel is uncertain, it seems probable that the ileum is affected as well as the jejunum.

5.3 Skin disease

The complex relationship between skin disease and intestinal malabsorption is sometimes a source of diagnostic confusion. It is well known that a variety of non-specific skin rashes may complicate primary intestinal disturbances, especially adult coeliac disease. Conversely, intestinal malabsorption, and even minor abnormalities of the jejunal mucosa, may be associated with skin disease such as psoriasis and eczema. In neither case has the mechanism underlying the relationship been clearly established (see Marks and Shuster, 1970). More easy to understand are conditions in which both skin and small bowel are affected by a systematized disease process. Progressive systemic sclerosis (Section 5.4) and allergic gastroenteropathy (Section 7.3) provide good examples of this kind of association. The rare hereditary condition acrodermatitis enteropathica, probably also falls into this category. A centrifugal dermatitis is often accompanied by malabsorption, and a patchy non-specific mucosal abnormality has been detected by jejunal biopsy (Ament and Broviac, 1973). Serum zinc levels have been found to be reduced, and clinical improvement follows oral diodoquin or zinc therapy. A distinctive ultrastructure abnormality is seen in the Paneth cell granules (Lombeck et al., 1974, Bohane et al., 1977).

From the diagnostic viewpoint, however, the well-recognized association between dermatitis herpetiformis (DH) and coeliac disease is of particular importance (Marks 1966). It is becoming apparent that in almost all patients with D. H. jejunal biopsy reveals mucosal abnormality of variable severity (Scott et al., 1976) and that the intestinal disturbance, and sometimes the skin disease, improve following the withdrawal of gluten from the diet (Fry et al., 1973). In D. H., it is notable that the functional and morphological expression of gluten sensitivity is often less well-developed than in the more typical forms of coeliac disease. Thus the finding of subtotal villous atrophy in a jejunal biopsy is the exception rather than the rule. Varying degrees of partial villous atrophy are more usual although any phase in the evolution of the mucosal lesion of coeliac disease can be encountered (Fig. 5.6). In some cases there may be little more than mild damage to the villous epithelium and an increase in intra-epithelial lymphocytes (Fig. 5.7). Another notable feature is the patchiness of the mucosal change, (Scott and Losowsky, 1976) which may differ not only between one biopsy and another but between different parts of the same biopsy (Fig. 5.8). No doubt this phenomenon accounts for the varying incidence of mucosal abnormality reported in studies of D. H. The higher incidence of the histocompatibility antigen HLA–8 observed in coeliac disease is also found in D. H. (Scott *et al.*, 1976). While these findings might indicate that some individuals inherit a genetic predisposition both to D. H. and to coeliac disease, it has recently been suggested that in coeliac disease mucosal damage generates circulating immune complexes which might be responsible for the skin lesions of D. H. as well

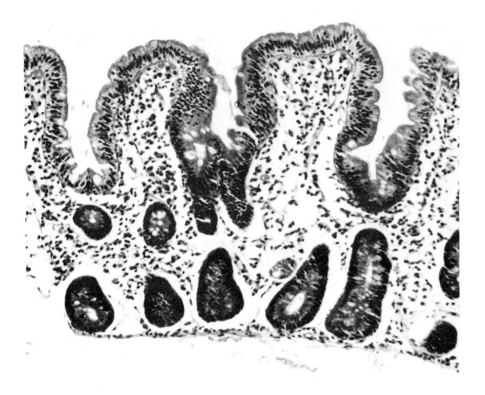

Fig. 5.6(a) Dermatitis herpetiformis. In this jejunal biopsy there is a moderate degree of partial villous atrophy. HE × 180.

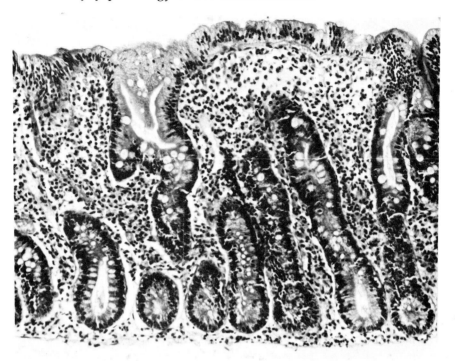

Fig. 5.6(b) Dermatitis herpetiformis. There is subtotal villous atrophy. This is same biopsy as represented in (a) illustrating the variability in the mucosal appearances. HE × 180.

as for a large variety of other immunological disturbances which may complicate this condition such as allergic alveolitis and rheumatoid arthritis (Scott and Losowsky, 1975).

5.4 The 'blind loop' syndrome (stasis syndrome)

The predominant factor in limiting bacterial proliferation in the lumen of the small bowel is the rapid transit time of the intestinal contents. Stasis, however produced, inevitably leads to abnormal bacterial growth. If sufficently prolonged it will result in a malabsorptive disturbance characterized mainly by vitamin B12 deficiency and steatorrhoea (see Badenoch *et al.*, 1955a).

Among the most important causes of stasis are surgical blind loops, including afferent loops produced by partial gastrectomy of the Polya type, jejunal diverticular disease and chronic small bowel obstruction. Less often, interference with intestinal motility by progressive sys-

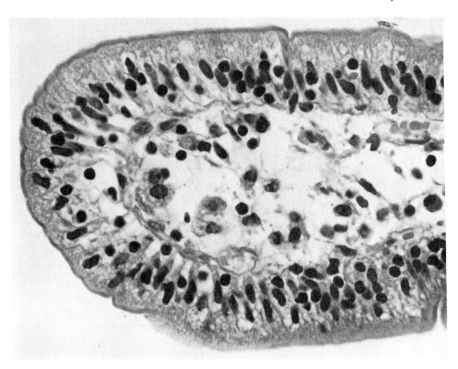

Fig. 5.7 Dermatitis herpetiformis. The only abnormalities in this case are an increase in intra-epithelial lymphocytes and mild enterocyte damage at the villous extremity. HE × 720.

temic sclerosis, by drugs such as ganglion-blocking agents and possibly by ionizing radiation can be blamed.

Exposure of the intestinal mucosa to abnormal bacterial growth leads to mucosal abnormality, the extent of which is co-terminous with the area exposed. This is particularly well illustrated in jejunal diverticular disease, in which the abnormal bacterial growth is largely confined to the lumina of diverticula. Outside the diverticula, the mucosal pattern is usually normal (Fig. 5.8); whereas within the diverticula, the mucosa shows crypt hyperplastic villous atrophy, which may be subtotal in some places (Fig. 5.9). Resected blind loops may also show villous atrophy, usually of the partial type (Fig. 4.45).

Thus, in most cases of malabsorption due to stasis, random proximal jejunal biopsy will reveal mucosal abnormality only in exceptional circumstances, although abnormal bacterial growth may be detected. On rare occasions for example, a biopsy might be taken from within a diverticulum. The varying degrees of villous atrophy reported in

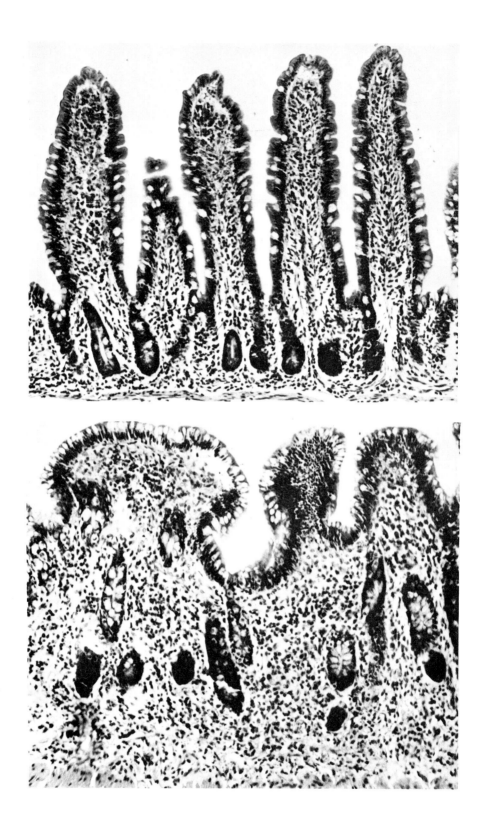

jejunal biopsies from some patients with Crohn's disease, however, may well be a consequence of intestinal stasis.

There is now evidence for a direct toxic effect of the unconjugated bile salts on the epithelium in stasis syndrome (Tabaqchali and Booth, 1966; Gracey *et al.*, 1973). While histologically there are few obvious abnormalities, the cells show more significant ultrastructural abnormalities than might be expected. Ament *et al.* (1972) in a study of three patients with stasis syndrome found fewer lipid particles than normal in the absorptive cells, fewer cells involved in fat absorption, and impairment of chylomicron transport to the lamina propria. Similar changes have been produced by experimentally induced stasis syndrome in animals, as well as by feeding or by intestinal perfusion of deconjugated bile salts. Parallel ultrastructural and histochemical abnormalities have been demonstrated in rats with self-filling blind loops (Gracey *et al.*, 1974); some abnormalities were found distal to, but not proximal to these loops. Self-emptying blind loops showed no changes (Toskes *et al.*, 1975).

5.5 Immune deficiency syndromes

Considering the importance of the small intestine as a lymphoid organ it is hardly surprising that disturbance of intestinal function or morphology may be a notable feature of the immune deficiency syndrome. Malabsorption appears to be especially associated with acquired forms of hypogammaglobulinaemia, the so-called 'hypogammaglobulinaemic sprue'. While the classification of hypogammaglobulinaemic syndromes is still in a state of some confusion, intestinal biopsy may provide valuable diagnostic information in such conditions. Of particular importance are the presence of large or abnormal lymphoid aggregates in the intestinal mucosa, and a deficiency of plasma cells in the lamina propria. The immunoperoxidase technique (Section 2.4) may also detect an abnormal distribution of immunoglobulin, or absence of a particular class of immunoglobulin, in the intestinal plasma cell population. Variable degrees of villous abnormality are found in a minority of cases. The following types of hypogammaglobulinaemia illustrate these points.

(a) *Severe generalized hypogammaglobulinaemia* Patients with severe

---

Fig. 5.8 Jejunal diverticulosis. The mucosa outside the diverticula is normal. HE × 180.

Fig. 5.9 Jejunal diverticulosis. The mucosa inside a diverticulum shows severe partial villous atrophy. This is the same case as is illustrated in Fig. 5.8. HE × 180.

generalized hypogammaglobulinaemia are especially prone to develop intestinal malabsorption. Jejunal biopsy presents a variable villous pattern and the subtotal villous atrophy occasionally found is similar to coeliac disease apart from a virtual absence of plasma cells. American workers hold the view that both the malabsorption and the villous abnormalities are due to giardiasis and respond to the appropriate drug therapy (Ament and Rubin, 1972). In similar cases reported from Britain, however, in which gluten withdrawal has produced a favourable response, the mucosal damage might well be due to complicating coeliac disease (see Asquith, 1974).

(b) *Sex-linked hypogammaglobulinaemia* In classical sex-linked hypogammaglobulinaemia jejunal biopsy usually shows a normal pattern although plasma cells are absent and the lymphoid aggregates lack germinal centres.

(c) *Selective IgA deficiency* Most individuals with selective IgA deficiency are healthy and the intestinal biopsy is normal, apart, of course, from a virtual absence of IgA-producing plasma cells. IgM-producing plasma cells appear to be capable of compensating for this deficit. Some IgA-deficient subjects however, develop coeliac disease with subtotal villous atrophy and show a typical response to gluten withdrawal (Asquith *et al.*, 1969). While it seems unlikely that the two conditions are causally related, it is notable that in two IgA-deficient patients with coeliac disease studied recently in Glasgow, rheumatoid arthritis was a complicating factor, and one patient had auto-immune haemolytic anaemia.

(d) *Nodular lymphoid hyperplasia* In one group of hypogammaglobulinaemic patients there is a marked reduction in the serum level of IgA and IgM with a variable depression of IgG, and jejunal biopsy shows abnormal prominence of the lymphoid aggregates. Measuring up to 4 mm in diameter, these structures consist histologically of ill-defined germinal centres with only a thin mantle of small lymphocytes (Fig. 4.31). This lesion is usually referred to as nodular lymphoid hyperplasia (Hermans *et al.*, 1966). In addition there is a virtual absence of plasma cells in the lamina propria, and giardiasis is an almost invariable complication (Fig. 4.30). While the villous pattern is commonly normal, partial villous atrophy is observed in some cases, possibly as a result of the giardiasis (Fig. 5.10). Cerainly malabsorption when present, which is by no means always the case, may respond to treatment of the giardia infestation (Ament and Rubin, 1972).

5.6 Gastric surgery

Malabsorption may be a troublesome complication of surgical pro-

cedures involving gastro-jejunal anastomosis, such as gastroenterostomy, or partial gastrectomy of the Polya type. It can usually be
attributed to disordered stimulation of pancreatic secretion or delayed
emptying of the gallbladder. Abnormal bacterial growth in the afferent
jejunal loop is occasionally responsible for impaired absorption of
vitamin B12 (Badenoch *et al.*, 1955b). Despite the alterations in the
luminal environment of the upper jejunum which follow such operations, there is little evidence of disturbed intestinal function. In the
majority of cases, biopsy studies have shown that intestinal morphology is normal (Scott *et al.*, 1964; Roy-Choudhury *et al.*, 1966).

However, in a small but important group of patients with post-
gastrectomy malabsorption, intestinal biopsy reveals subtotal villous
atrophy. This is almost always due to clinically unsuspected coeliac
disease (Section 5.1). In such cases it seems likely that the surgical
procedure has been sufficient to 'activate' a previously dormant intestinal disease process (Lee, 1970). Evidence for this is provided
by the occasional presence of crypt irregularity, crypt abscess formation and pyloric metaplasia, all of which are markers of an ulcerative
process not usually seen in coeliac disease (Fig. 5.4). Since similar
changes are seen in the immediate vicinity of stomal ulcers, it seems
probable that they are caused by high acid levels in the jejunum
(see below). Whether such chemical alterations alone can ever produce a true subtotal villous atrophy in the jejunum remains uncertain
although operative resections have occasionally shown patchy atrophic
change (Paulley *et al.*, 1957; Fig. 5.11), and in the Zollinger-Ellison
syndrome, in which an exceptionally high acid output by the stomach
is provoked by the presence of a gastrin-secreting tumour, patchy
villous atrophy of variable severity has been observed in the jejunum
(Singleton *et al.*, 1965). Atrophic changes seen in 'ileal bladders' are
presumably also due to chemical effects (Townley *et al.*, 1964). Thus it
may not be possible on morphological grounds to make a clear distinction between coeliac disease and 'chemical effect' in a random biopsy.
In this case, only the clinical response to a gluten-free diet will settle
the matter.

The detection of recurrent peptic ulceration at the gastro-jejunal
stoma is largely a clinical or radiological problem. Nonetheless, as
mentioned above, operative resections often reveal mucosal changes,
only rarely seen in random intestinal biopsies, including pyloric metaplasia and crypt abscess formation. They are usually associated with
the localized hypertrophic villous pattern described in Section 4.2.2
and are essentially pre-ulcerative or post-ulcerative in nature.

Finally, a diffuse hypoplastic villous pattern, associated with 'dwarf
villi' and equally diminutive crypts (Fig. 4.48), is occasionally seen in

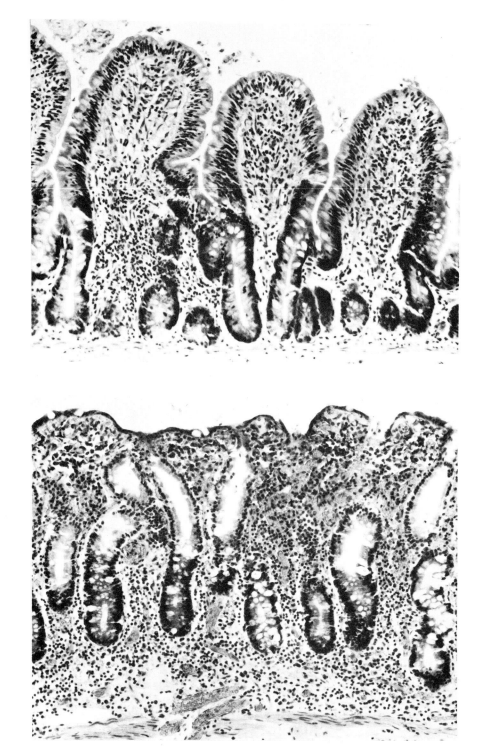

patients suffering from severe malnutrition after gastric surgery. This state is due mainly to diminished food intake, possibly exacerbated by malabsorption. It seems likely that the mucosal alteration is simply caused by reduced functional demand (Section 4.2.3).

5.7 Malignant tumours

Mucosal changes are commonly seen in the immediate vicinity of malignant intestinal tumours, regardless of their histogensis (Lee, 1966). Such *localized* changes, quantitatively similar to those found around other gross ulcerative lesions, correspond histologically to the 'hypertrophic' villous pattern described in Section 4.2.2, and have little functional significance. Occasionally, however, malignant tumours are accompanied by *diffuse* mucosal changes, usually taking the form of partial or subtotal villous atrophy. These are particularly found in association with the malignant lymphoid tumours. In most instances it seems probable that such diffuse atrophic changes are due to pre-existing coeliac disease, since it is now thought that this disease predisposes to the development of neoplasia, especially primary malignant lymphoma of the upper small intestine (Gough *et al.*, 1962). There also appears to be an increased incidence of carcinoma in other parts of the alimentary system, particularly the oesophagus, and possibly of neoplasia outside the alimentary tract, such as nodal Hodgkin's disease (see Harris *et al.*, 1967). Hodgkin's disease only rarely affects the gut itself in C.D.; more often it arises in mesenteric or even in peripheral lymph nodes. Curiously enough, carcinoma of the small bowel only rarely complicates coeliac disease.

These observations provide an explanation for the occasional finding of villous atrophy in jejunal biopsies taken from patients suffering not only from a variety of intestinal neoplasms but also from extra-intestinal malignancy (see Hindle and Creamer, 1965). The special risk of lymphoma in coeliac disease is such that attempts have been made to predict the onset of this complication from analysis of the leucocytic infiltrate in the lamina propria in random jejunal biopsies (Ferguson *et al.*, 1974; see Section 5.1).

Fig. 5.10 Hypogammaglobulinaemia. There is partial villous atrophy, probably caused by complicating giardiasis. This patient also had nodular lymphoid hyperplasia. HE × 180.
Fig. 5.11 Gastrojejunostomy. The mucosa in the afferent jejunal loop shows subtotal villous atrophy. In this case, frank ulceration was present at the stoma, and the villous pattern was normal in the distal resected end of the afferent loop. HE × 180.

In some cases of intestinal neoplasia with diffuse villous atrophy, it is difficult to prove that coeliac disease is responsible for the mucosal changes. Malabsorption is commonly absent, and when present may be of short duration or unresponsive to gluten withdrawal despite severe and extensive mucosal damage (Figs. 5.12 and 5.13). These patients are often in late middle age and give no history of previous intestinal disturbance. Whether in such cases the mucosal atrophy is due to atypical or asymptomatic coeliac disease, or is in some way provoked by the presence of a malignant intestinal tumour, remains a matter for speculation. The important lesson is that when jejunal biopsy reveals villous atrophy which cannot be readily explained, or shows an atypical leucocytic infiltrate in the lamina propria mucosae, the possibility of intestinal neoplasia should be seriously considered, especially if the patient is beyond middle age.

5.8 Malnutrition

There is evidence from both human and experimental sources that nutritional disturbances can produce morphological change in the intestinal mucosa. Perhaps the best documented example of this in human pathology is the serious form of protein deficiency found all too often in children in tropical developing countries and known in Africa as kwashiorkor. During the active phase of this disease the jejunal mucosa may appear completely 'flat' under the dissecting microscope and presents the histological features of crypt hyperplastic subtotal villous atrophy; (Stanfield et al., 1965). Such villi as can be measured are reduced in height, even by tropical standards, the crypt-to-villus ratio is increased and there is increased leucocytic infiltration in the lamina propria. The presence of abnormalities in the villous epithelial cells enhances the similarity to coeliac disease (Section 4.1.2), although there are some quantitative differences, in particular the pronounced reduction in Paneth cells regularly observed in kwashiorkor (Trowell et al., 1954). An improvement in the nutritional status leads to marked improvement in mucosal morphology, (Cook and Lee, 1966) but even so, a possible explanation for the villous changes in kwashiorkor may lie in transient gluten sensitivity. In fatal cases of kwashiorkor, the crypt hyperplasia observed during earlier phases of the disease

---

Fig.5.12 Intestinal lymphoma. The mucosa shows diffuse partial villous atrophy. There is a marked increase in lymphocytes both in the lamina propria and within the villous epithelium. HE × 180.

Fig. 5.13 Intestinal lymphoma. A high power view of the mucosa illustrated in Fig. 5.12 showing the striking increase in intra-epithelial lymphocytes. HE × 720.

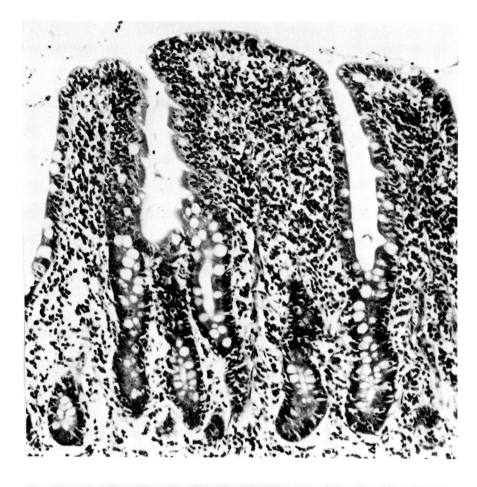

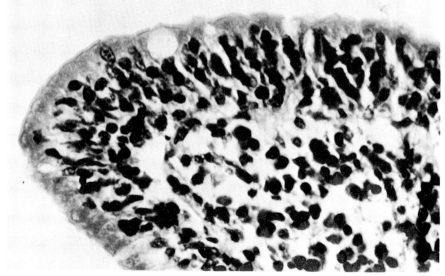

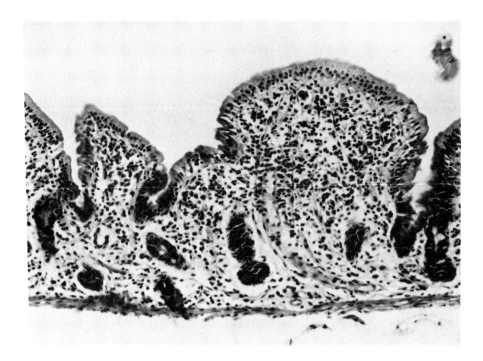

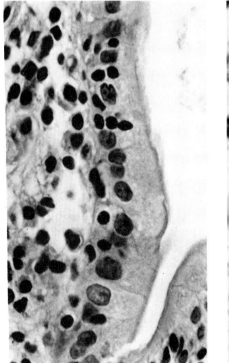
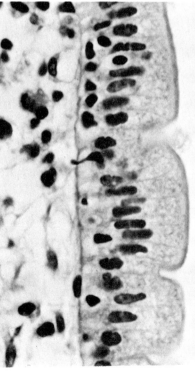

becomes less pronounced, nuclear abnormalities appear in the regenerative crypt cells (Fig. 4.12) and a severe state of hypoplastic villous atrophy supervenes (Section 4.2.3; Fig. 4.49), consistent with the finding in experimental animals (see below).

Malnutrition of a degree comparable to kwashiorkor is seldom observed in developed countries. Less severe forms are, however, not uncommon, such as in patients with debilitating disease (Creamer, 1965) or following gastric surgery. Reduced food intake is the usual cause. In such instances, the jejunal mucosa may show mild hypoplastic villous atrophy, with reduction in villous height associated with a proportional fall in crypt height (Fig. 4.48, see Section 4.2.3). The appearances resemble those observed experimentally in protein-deficient mice (Deo and Ramalingaswami, 1965) and are presumably due to defective output of enterocytes from the crypts of Lieberkuhn. Hypoplastic mucosal abnormalities, sometimes associated with megalocytic changes in developing enterocytes, have also been observed in some cases of vitamin B12 deficiency (Whitehead, 1971) and folate deficiency (Figs. 5.14 and 5.15). This is a curious finding. In the haemopoietic system, vitamin B12 or folic acid deficiency results in defective output of red cells, but there is marked marrow hyperplasia, mainly due to delayed maturation of developing red cells, many of which die within the marrow ('ineffective erythropoiesis'). By analogy, one would expect pronounced hyperplasia of the crypts of Lieberkühn to be a notable feature of B12 or folate deficiency, which is not usually the case, except possibly in children with folate deficiency. (Davidson and Townley, 1977.)

References

Adlersberg, D. and Schein, J. (1947), Clinical and pathologic studies in sprue. *J. Am. med. Ass.*, **134**, 1459–1467.

Ament, M. and Rubin, C. E. (1972), Relation of giardiasis to abnormal intestinal structure and function in gastrointestinal immunodeficiency syndromes. *Gastroenterology*, **62**, 216–226.

Ament, M. and Rubin, C. E. (1972b), Soy protein – another cause of the flat intestinal lesion. *Gastroenterology*, **62**, 227–234.

Ament, M., Shimoda, S. S., Saunders, D. R. and Rubin, C. E. (1972), Pathogenesis of steatorrhoea in three cases of small intestinal stasis syndrome. *Gastroenterology*, **63**, 728–747.

Fig. 5.14 Folate deficiency. There is severe villous atrophy of crypt hypoplastic type. The serum folate level was 0.1 ng ml.$^{-1}$ HE $\times$ 180.

Fig. 5.15 Folate deficiency. In this composite picture the macrocytic villous epithelium in a folate-deficient patient (left) is compared with normal villous epithelium (right). HE $\times$ 815.

Ament, M. and Broviac, J. (1973), Acrodermatitis enteropathica. Demonstration of small and large intestinal mucosal lesions: failure of hyperalimentation, intralipid and Diodoquin to reverse the intestinal lesions and generalized malabsorption syndrome. *Gastroenterology*, **64**, 692. (Abstract)

Asquith, P., Thompson, R. A. and Cooke, W. T. (1969), Serum immunoglobulins in adult coeliac disease. *Lancet*, **2**, 129–131.

Asquith, P. (1974), Immunology. In *Clinics in Gastroenterology 3, No. 1 (Coeliac disease)*, p. 213. Saunders, London.

Badenoch, J., Bedford, R. D. and Evans, J. R. (1955a), Massive diverticulosis of the small intestine with steatorrhoea and megaloblastic anaemia. *Q. J. Med.*, **24**, 321–330.

Badenoch, J., Evans, J. R., Richards, W. C. D. and Witts, L. J. (1955b), Megaloblastic anaemia following partial gastrectomy and gastroenterostomy. *Br. J. Haemat.*, **1**, 339–344.

Baker, S. J., Ignatius, M., Mathan, V. I., Vaish, S. K. and Chacko, C. C. (1962), Tropical sprue. In *Intestinal Biopsy. Ciba Foundation Study Group No. 14*, (Ed. Wolstenholme, G. E. W. and Cameron, M. P.), pp. 84–101. Churchill, London.

Banwell, J. G. and Gorbach, S. L. (1969), Tropical sprue. *Gut*, **10**. 328–333.

Barry, R. E., Morris, J. S. and Read, A. E. (1970), A case of small intestinal mucosal atrophy. *Gut*, **11**, 743–747.

Bayless, T. M., Kapelowitz, R. F., Shelley, W. M., Ballinger, W. F. and Hendrix, T. R. (1967), Intestinal ulceration – a complication of coeliac disease. *N. Engl. J. Med.*, **276**, 996–1002.

Bohane, T. D., Cutz, E., Hamilton, J. R. and Gall, D. G. (1977), Acrodermatitis enteropathica, zinc and the Paneth cell. A case report with family studies. *Gastroenterology*, **73**, 587–592.

Bossart, R., Henry, K., Booth, C. C. and Doe, W. F. (1975), Collagenous basement membrane thickening in jejunal biopsies from patients with adult coeliac disease. *Gut*, **15**, 338. (Abstract)

Brunser, O., Eidelman, S. and Klipstein, F. A. (1970), Intestinal mucosa of rural Haitians. A comparison between overt tropical sprue and asymptomatic subjects. *Gastroenterology*, **58**, 655–668.

Butterworth, C. E. Jr. and Perez-Santiago, E. (1958), Pathologic changes in jejunal biopsies from sprue patients. *Ann. intern. Med.*, **48**, 8–29.

Challacombe, D. N., Dawkins, P. D., Baylis, J. M. and Robertson, K. (1975), Small intestinal histology in coeliac disease. *Lancet*, **1**, 1345–1346 (letter).

Cook, G. C. and Lee, F. D. (1966), The jejunum after Kwashiorkor. *Lancet*, **2**, 1263–1267.

Creamer, B. (1965), The dynamics of the small intestinal mucosa. In *Recent Advances in Gastroenterology* (Ed. Badenoch, J. and Brooke, B. N.), pp. 148–161. Little, Brown and Co., Boston.

Davidson, G. P. and Townley, R. R. W. (1977), Structural and functional abnormalities of the small intestine due to intestinal folic acid deficiency in infancy. *J. Pediat.*, **90**, 590–594.

Deo, M. G. and Ramalingaswami, V. (1965), Reaction of the small intestine to induced protein malnutrition in Rhesus monkeys – a study of cell population kinetics in the jejunum. *Gastroenterology*, **49**, 150–157.

Falchuk, Z. M., Rogentine, G. N. and Strober, W. (1972), Predominance of histocompatibility antigen HLA-8 in patients with gluten-sensitive enteropathy. *J. clin. Invest.*, **51**, 1602–1605.

Ferguson, A. and Murray, D. (1977), Quantitation of intraepithelial lymphocytes in human jejunum. *Gut*, **12**, 988–994.

Ferguson, R., Asquith, P. and Cooke, W. T. (1974), The jejunal cellular infiltrate in coeliac disease complicated by lymphoma. *Gut*, **15**, 458–461.

Fry, L., Seah, P. P., Riches, D. J. and Hoffbrand, A. V. (1973), Clearance of skin lesions in dermatitis herpetiformis after gluten withdrawal. *Lancet*, **1**, 288–291.

Gough, K. R., Read, A. E. and Naish, J. M. (1962), Intestinal reticulosis as a complication of idiopathic steatorrhoea. *Gut*, **3**, 232–239.

Gorbach, S. L., Banwell, J. G., Mitra, R., Chatterjee, B. D., Jacobs, B. and Mazumder, D. N. G. (1969), Bacterial contamination of the upper small bowel in tropical sprue. *Lancet*, **1**, 74–77.

Gracey, M., Papadimitriou, J., Burke, V., Thomas, J. and Bower, G. (1973), Effects on small intestinal function and structure induced by feeding a deconjugated bile salt. *Gut*, **14**, 519–528.

Gracey, M., Papadimitriou, J. and Bower, G. (1974), Ultrastructural changes in the small intestines of rats with self-filling blind loops. *Gastroenterology*, **67**, 646–651.

Harris, O. D., Cooke, W. T., Thompson, H. and Waterhouse, J. A. H. (1967), Malignancy in adult coeliac disease and idiopathic steatorrhoea. *Am. J. Med.*, **42**, 899–912.

Hermans, R. E., Huizenga, K. A., Hoffman, H. W., Brown, A. L. Snr. and Markowitz, H. (1966), Dysgammaglobulinaemia associated with nodular lymphoid hyperplasia of the small intestine. *Am. J. Med.*, **40,** 78–79.

Hindle, W. and Creamer, B. (1965), Significance of a flat small intestinal mucosa. *Br. med. J.*, **2**, 455–459.

Jeffries, G. H., Steinberg, H. and Sleisenger, M. H. (1968), Chronic ulcerative (non-granulomatous) jejunitis. *Am. J. Med.*, **44**, 47–59.

Lee, F. D. (1966), The nature of the mucosal changes associated with malignant tumours of the small intestine. *Gut*, **7**, 361–367.

Lee, F. D. (1970), *The intestinal mucosa in health and disease.* M.D. Thesis, University of Dundee.

Lombeck, I., von Bassewitz, D. B., Becker, K., Tinschamann, P. and Kastner, H. (1974). Ultrastructural findings in acrodermatitis enteropathica. *Pediat. Res.*, **8**, 82–88.

Marks, J., Shuster, M. and Watson, A. J. (1966), Small bowel changes in dermatitis herpetiformis. *Lancet*, **2**, 1280–1282.

Marks, J. and Shuster, S. (1970), Small intestinal mucosal abnormalities in various skin diseases – fact or fancy? *Gut*, **11**, 281–291.

Marsh, M. N. (1972), The scanning electron microscope and its application to the investigation of intestinal structure. In *Recent Advances in Gastroenterology*, (Ed. Badenoch, J. and Brooke, B. N.), 2nd Edition. Churchill Livingstone, Edinburgh.

Marsh, M. N., Brown. A. C. and Swift, J. A. (1970), The surface ultrastructure of the small intestinal mucosa of normal control human subjects and of patients with untreated and treated coeliac disease using the scanning electron microscope. In *Coeliac Disease*. (Ed. Booth, C. C. and Dowling, R. H.). Churchill Livingstone, London.

Mason, K. E. and Telford, I. R. (1947), Some manifestations of vitamin E deficiency in the monkey. *Archs. Path.*, **43**, 363–373.

Paulley, J. W., Fairweather, F. A. and Leeming, A. (1957), Post-gastrectomy steatorrhoea and patchy jejunal atrophy. *Lancet*, **1**, 406–407.

Pink, I. J. and Creamer, B. (1967), Response to a gluten free diet of patients with coeliac syndrome. *Lancet*, **1**, 300–304.

Roy-Choudhury, D., Cooke, W. T., Tan, D. T., Banwell, J. G. and Smits, B. J. (1966), Jejunal biopsy: criteria and significance. *Scand. J. Gastroenterol.*, **1**, 57–74.

Schwartz, M. and Jarnum, S. (1959), Gastrointestinal protein loss in idiopathic (hypercatabolic) hypoproteinaemia. *Lancet*, **1**, 327–330.

Scott, G. B., Williams, M. J. and Clark, C. G. (1964), Comparison of jejunal mucosa in post-gastrectomy states, idiopathic steatorrhoea and controls using the dissecting microscope and conventional histological methods. *Gut*, **5**, 553–562.

Scott, B. B. and Losowsky, M. (1975), Coeliac disease: a cause of various associated diseases? *Lancet*, **2**, 956–957.

Scott, B. B. and Losowsky, M. S. (1976), Patchiness and duodenal-jejunal variation of the mucosal abnormality in coeliac disease and dermatitis herpetiformis. *Gut*, **17**, 984–992.

Scott, B. B., Young, S., Rajah, S. M., Marks, J. and Losowsky, M. S. (1976), Coeliac disease and dermatitis herpetiformis: further studies of their relationship. *Gut*, **17**, 759–762.

Sheehy, T. W. and Perez-Santiago, E. (1961), Antibiotic therapy in tropical sprue. *Gastroenterology*, **41**, 208–214.

Sheehy, T. W., Baggs, B., Perez-Santiago, E. and Floch, M. H. (1962), Prognosis of tropical sprue. A study of the effect of folic acid on the intestinal aspects of acute and chronic sprue. *Ann. intern. Med.*, **57**, 892–908.

Shiner, M., Ballard, J., Brook, C. G. D., Herman, S. and Lovell, D. (1975), Jejunal biopsy in the management of infants suspected of cow's milk protein intolerance. *Gut*, **16**, 822. (Abstract)

Singleton, J. W., Kern, F. and Waddell, W. R. (1965), Diarrhea and pancreatic islet cell tumour. Report of a case with severe jejunal mucosal lesion. *Gastroenterology*, **49**, 197–208.

Stanfield, J. P., Hutt, M. S. R. and Tunnicliffe, R. (1956), Intestinal biopsy in Kwashiorkor. *Lancet*, **2**, 519–523.

Swanson, V. L. and Thomassen, D. V. M. (1965), Pathology of the jejunal mucosa in tropical sprue. *Am. J. Path.*, **46**, 511–551.

Tabaqchali, S. and Booth, C. C. (1966), Jejunal bacteriology and bile-salt metabolism in patients with intestinal malabsorption. *Lancet*, **2**, 12–15.

Thomas, G. and Clain, D. J. (1976), Endemic tropical sprue in Rhodesia. *Gut*, **17**, 877–887.

Toskes, P. P., Gianella, R. A., Jervis, H. R., Rout, W. R. and Takeuchi, A. (1975), Small intestinal mucosal injury in the experimental blind loop syndrome. Light and electron microscopic and histochemical studies. *Gastroenterology*, **68**, 1193–1203.

Townley, R. R. W., Cass, M. H. and Anderson, C. M. (1964), Small intestinal mucosal patterns of coeliac disease and idiopathic steatorrhoea seen in other situations. *Gut*, **5**, 51–55.

Trowell, H. C., Davies, J. N. P. and Dean, R. F. A. (1954), In *Kwashiorkor*, pp. 149–150. Edward Arnold, London.

Ward, M. Eastwood, M. A. and Ferguson, A. (1976), Jejunal lysozyme and Paneth cell population in coeliac disease. *Gut*, **17**, 813. (Abstract)

Weinstein, W., Saunders, D., Tytgat, G. and Rubin, C. E. (1970), Collagenous sprue – an unrecognized type of malabsorption. *N. Engl. J. Med.*, **283**, 1297–1301.

Whitehead, R. (1971), The interpretation and significance of morphological abnormalities in jejunal biopsies. In *Intestinal Absorption and its Derangements* (Ed. Dawson, A. M.), *J. clin. Path.*, **24**, Suppl. (Roy. Coll. Path.) **5**, 108–124.

6 Malabsorptive states with distinctive pathological changes

This section is concerned with a small but select group of disease states which can be accurately diagnosed by random intestinal biopsy. While multisystem involvement is observed in most of the conditions in this group, intestinal malabsorption is often an important if not a presenting feature, and histological abnormalities which are both diffuse and distinctive are invariably present in the intestinal mucosa or submucosa.

6.1 Whipple's disease

This rare and curious disease, which predominantly affects middle-aged males, has been a subject of recurrent interest since it was first described in 1907 (Whipple, 1907). While intestinal disturbance is usually pre-eminent both clinically and pathologically, multisystem involvement is well recognized. Symptoms such as arthralgia, fever and chronic cough may precede those related to the intestinal tract and to impaired absorption. Distinctive pathological changes have been described in many organs including lymph nodes, heart valves, central nervous system, spleen, lungs, liver, kidneys and endocrine glands (Farnan, 1965). It is, however, from the histological appearances of the intestinal mucosa – especially the jejunum – that the diagnosis is usually made, and the changes are sufficiently diffuse to be detectable by random biopsy in most cases (see also Section 4.1.3).

The characteristic feature is an infiltration of histiocytes the cytoplasm of which is swollen by the presence of numerous faintly eosinophilic, P.A.S. - positive granules (Fig. 4.26): the infiltrate is seen initially and is always most prominent in the lamina propria, especially at the villous extremity, although some overspill into the submucosa is occasionally seen. Stainable iron may be detected in both mucosal and submucosal histiocytes. This is a curious finding, since there is often an iron-deficiency anaemia with low serum iron levels (Hourihane, 1966). A similar phenomenon is found in rheumatoid arthritis, especially in the presence of amyloidosis (Section 6.4). Neutrophil polymorphs may also be found in the lamina propria, particularly at the villous extremity (Fig. 6.1) or at a deeper level surrounding the characteristic clear spaces (Fig. 4.26). Some of these spaces – which can be shown in frozen section to contain a neutral fat – have a distinct endothelial lining and may represent dilated lacteals. The 'normal' population of leucocytes in the lamina propria is seldom conspicuous but can still be detected: probably it is 'pushed aside' rather than replaced by the abnormal histiocytic infiltrate.

Epithelial damage is not a notable feature of Whipple's disease; the intestinal brush border is usually entirely normal. The villi are of course greatly distended by histiocytic accumulation (Fig. 6.2) and a flat mucosal appearance resembling 'pseudo-atrophy' (Section 4.2.2) is quite common. This latter appearance is probably due to fusion of swollen villi rather than to any disturbance of enterocyte dynamics, and it is notable that dilated crypts, clearly occluded by epithelial adhesions, can sometimes be observed.

The histological diagnosis of Whipple's disease seldom presents serious difficulty, at least in a jejunal biopsy. Of course, the other causes of histiocytic infiltration in the lamina propria (Section 4.1.3) have to be excluded, and it has to be remembered that the occasional histiocyte with P.A.S.-positive cytoplasmic granules can be found at the villous extremity under normal conditions. The possibility of a misdiagnosis is much greater in biopsies of the large intestine – which is occasionally involved in the disease process – since foamy histiocytes are invariably present and may be quite numerous in the lamina propria of the colonic mucosa even in normal individuals. These 'colonic histiocytes' are P.A.S.-positive but, unlike the abnormal histiocytes in Whipple's disease, are also mucicarminophilic and have sometimes been referred to as 'muciphages' (Arapakis and Tribe, 1962); they tend to be conspicuous in association with melanosis coli – indeed the same histiocytes may contain both mucin and pigment – and in some types of colonic dysfunction in young women ('colonic histiocytosis'; Pittman et al., 1966).

The nature of Whipple's disease is still uncertain. It now seems clear, however, that bacterial infection is an important factor in the pathogenesis of the disease. The administration of broad-spectrum antibiotics not only produces clinical improvement (Chears and Ashworth, 1961), but brings about a striking reduction in the histiocytic infiltrate in the intestinal mucosa. The cytoplasmic P.A.S.-positive

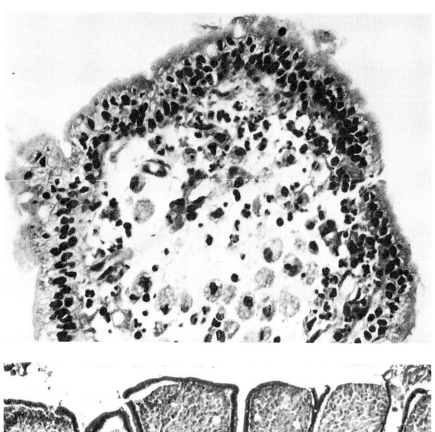
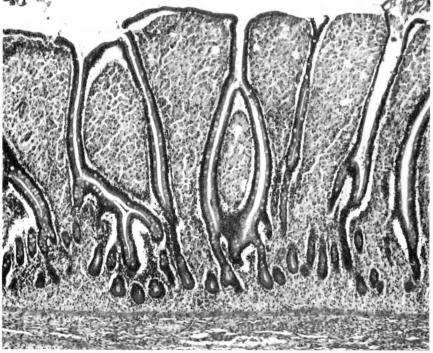

material within the abnormal histiocytes is, moreover, now thought to be a neutral polysaccharide or glycoprotein derived from bacterial cell walls (Yardley and Hendrix, 1961). The most convincing evidence for this comes mainly from electron microscopic studies (Section 4.1.3), which reveal numerous rod-shaped organisms in the tissues of the lamina propria in untreated cases. The macrophages ingest these in large phagolysosomes, where they are partially degraded. Residual undigested material, however, persists, forming the P.A.S.-positive inclusions of the macrophages. On treatment the free organisms rapidly disappear but the abnormal histiocytes may remain for a considerable period. Clinical relapse can be shown to correlate with the reappearance of free bacterial forms (Morningstar, 1975).

6.2 Abetalipoproteinaemia (Acanthocytosis or Bassen-Kornzweig Syndrome)

This rare, genetically determined disease is apparently inherited as an autosomal recessive (Salt et al., 1960) and is mostly confined to individuals of Jewish or Mediterranean descent. While the exact biochemical abnormality has yet to be elucidated, the principal disturbance is an inability to synthesise chylomicrons and other low-density lipoproteins. The pathological effects of this are most readily detected in the peripheral blood and intestinal tract, both of which may be involved from an early stage in life; neurological disturbance, characteristically taking the form of cerebellar ataxia, and atypical retinitis pigmentosa are not usually evident until adolescent or adult life.

The typical microscopic abnormality of the peripheral blood is a peculiar spiny deformation of the red cells – hence the term 'acanthocytosis' (Fig. 6.3). This may be associated with a slight reduction in red cell survival, although haemolytic anaemia is seldom found. The red cell change is thought to be due to an alteration in the membrane lipoprotein pattern, but is not morphologically specific; acanthocytosis has also been described in association with other hereditary neurological abnormalities.

The histological changes in the jejunal mucosa are, however, virtually diagnostic. While there is no significant disturbance of villous

---

Fig. 6.1 Whipple's disease. The lamina propria of the jejunal mucosa is infiltrated by histiocytes with granular, eosinophilic cytoplasm. Neutrophil polymorphs are also quite conspicuous in this case. HE × 450.
Fig. 6.2 Whipple's disease. A low-power view of the mucosa showing marked villous distension as a consequence of histiocytic infiltration of the lamina propria. There is also commencing villous fusion. HE × 85.

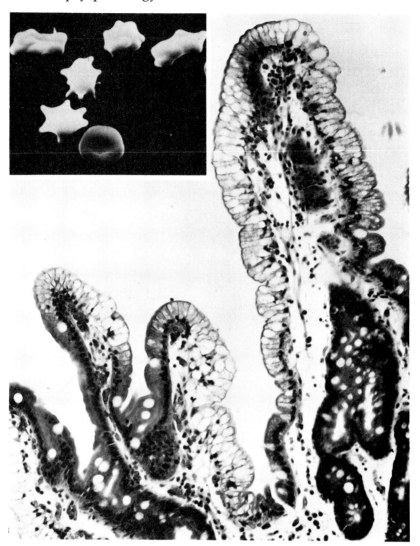

Fig. 6.3 Abetalipoproteinaemia. There is marked vacuolation and distension of the enterocytes at the villous extremity. The villous pattern is however normal. HE × 225. The insert (top left) shows the spiny deformity of the red cells (acanthocytosis) characteristic of the condition. SEM by courtesy of Dr K. E. Carr.

architecture (Lamy *et al.*, 1963) or enterocyte dynamics, the enterocytes reaching maturity towards the villous extremity invariably show pronounced cytoplasmic vacuolation (Fig. 6.3) which in frozen sections is seen to be due to presence of neutral fat. Initially, the fat globules are finely divided and give the enterocytes a foamy appearance; later the globules coalesce to produce cytoplasmic 'ballooning' (Fig. 4.7). Electron microscopy also presents a characteristic picture: the cells have a normal brush border and contain numerous fat droplets and increased numbers of lysosomes, which contain membranous components, myelin-like figures, lipid and paracrystalline material. Lipid is not found in the Golgi System, and there is an absence of chylomicrons in the basal intercellular spaces and the lamina propria. These features support the hypothesis of a defect in the transport mechanisms for removing fat from the absorptive cell. (Fig. 4.8; Dobbins, 1966; Kayden, 1972).

Vacuolation of enterocytes is quite often seen in other conditions, especially coeliac disease and tropical sprue, but is almost always associated with the atrophic villous pattern (Section 4.2.1). Moreover even in mild or early coeliac disease without gross architectural disturbance, cytoplasmic vacuolation is associated with other changes such as reduction in cell height and loss of nuclear polarity (Fig. 4.5), not to mention an increase in intra-epithelial lymphocytes and inflammatory changes in the lamina propria.

6.3 Intestinal lymphangiectasia

When this term is used in an unqualified sense it usually refers, as it does here, to a rare and probably congenital disease arising in the early years of life and attributable to an obstructive abnormality of the abdominal lymphatic system with extensive and pronounced dilatation of the lymphatics of the intestinal mucosa and submucosa. This is almost always part of a more generalized disturbance of lymphatic drainage, and asymmetrical oedema due to malformed lymphatics in one or other of the extremities is a common clinical finding (Mistilis *et al.*, 1965).

The disturbance of lymphatic drainage from the intestinal mucosa has several interesting functional consequences, the most notable of which is loss of protein into the intestinal lumen ('protein-losing enteropathy'; Waldmann, 1966). When the synthetic capacity of the body fails to compensate for this loss, hypoproteinaemia (involving all the major plasma protein components) and oedema inevitably develop. In a similar fashion there may be enteric loss of lymphocytes, and this is associated with a lymphopenia in the peripheral blood. Not surprisingly, the combination of lymphocyte depletion and hypogammaglobulinaemia predisposes to recurrent infection and defective cell-mediated immune responses have been reported (Strober *et al.*, 1967). As might be expected malabsorption of fat is a further consequence of lymphatic stasis, but it is not invariable and is seldom severe.

Random intestinal biopsy usually reveals a characteristic histological appearance, with extensive and pronounced dilatation of mucosal and submucosal lymphatic channels.

In the mucosa this results in marked villous distension (Fig. 6.4), responsible for the resemblance of the mucosal surface to a pebble beach under the dissecting microscope. Sometimes the villi are distorted and even appear to undergo fusion, although there is no evidence of a disturbance of enterocyte dynamics, despite the presence in some reported cases of pronounced intercellular oedema of the villous epithelium (Mistilis et al., 1965). In the submucosa, interstitial oedema may be conspicuous. Fat-laden histiocytes (lipophages) are commonly found both within lymphatic lumina and lying free in the interstices of the lamina propria and submucosa (Fig. 6.5). There may also be a slight non-specific inflammatory response (see Section 4.1.3) in the mucosa and, on occasion, a more acute response with neutrophil emigration into the epithelium of distended villi is found. The only other finding of importance is the presence of lipofuscin pigmentation of the intestinal smooth muscle: this is probably related to enteric protein loss and subsequent hypoalbuminaemia (Section 4.1.3), although it is not invariably present.

The histological features of intestinal lymphangiectasia are not entirely specific, and can be mimicked to some extent by any cause of extensive intestinal lymphatic occlusion or stasis. Interstitial oedema and lymphatic dilatation of variable degree may, for example, be found in congestive cardiac failure, constrictive pericarditis, retroperitoneal fibrosis and widespread mesenteric involvement with tumour (especially lymphoma) or tuberculosis (Rubin and Dobbins, 1965). In mesenteric tuberculosis, massive lipophage accumulation in the intestinal submucosa has been personally observed. Similar lymphatic changes have been observed in some disease processes directly affecting the intestinal wall, such as systemic sclerosis, radiation enteritis and Crohn's disease (Fig. 4.32). Mucosal lymphangiectasia may also be seen in association with dense interstitial deposits of hyalin material in Waldenstrom's macroglobulinaemia (Pruzanski et al., 1973). The lipophage accumulation observed in the mucosa and submucosa in the

Fig. 6.4 Intestinal lymphangiectasia. There is marked villous distension and dilatation of the villous lymphatic channels. HE × 105.

Fig. 6.5 Intestinal lymphangiectasia. Lipophages are found in the interstitial tissues of the jejunal submucosa close to dilated lymphatic channels, which contain similar cells. HE × 720.

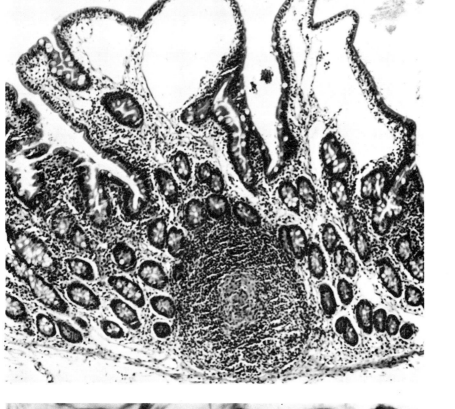

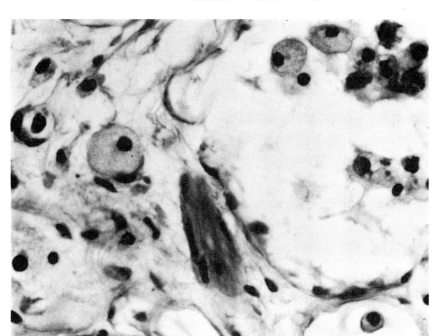

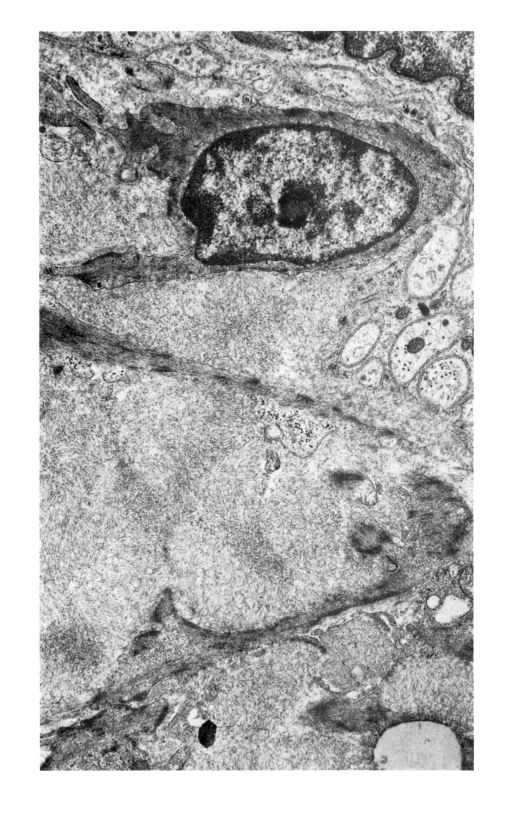

vicinity of jejunal diverticula may be due to lymphatic obstruction at the diverticular neck (Lee, 1966). Only rarely in such acquired conditions is the lymphatic dilatation in the mucosa as pronounced as it is in 'congenital' intestinal lymphangiectasia. In the unlikely event of a simple lymphangioma or lymphangiectatic cyst (Section 9.1) being included in a random intestinal biopsy, some difficulty may be encountered in distinguishing this lesion histologically from intestinal lymphangiectasia. A lymphangioma is, however, a purely localized lesion with dilatation of mucosal and submucosal lymphatics producing focal villous distortion (Fig. 9.1); the surrounding villi are normal. The dilated lymphatics may contain inspissated material and foamy histiocytes, but histiocytes are not conspicuous in the interstitial tissues (Shilken *et al.*, 1968); lipofuscinosis of the smooth muscle, is, moreover, absent, as are the other functional consequences of intestinal lymphangiectasia.

6.4 Intestinal amyloidosis

Amyloid disease, whether of the 'primary' or 'secondary' variety, commonly affects the intestinal tract and may be associated with a variety of clinical disturbances such as intractable diarrhoea, ischaemic damage, haemorrhage and perforation (Bero, 1957; Akbarian and Fenton, 1964). Malabsorption is also a well-recognized complication, but is decidely rare (Golden, 1954). In two personally studied cases of intestinal amyloidosis secondary to rheumatoid arthritis, there was non-specific superficial ulceration in the distal ileum, leading to recurrent haemorrhage and iron-deficiency anaemia. Despite this last finding, the histiocytes in the intestinal mucosa contained massive amounts of haemosiderin, presumably derived from orally administered iron, and the appearances suggested a defect in histiocytic function interfering with iron assimilation (Lee *et al.*, 1978). Whether this defect was in any way related to amyloidosis is uncertain; even so, mucosal haemosiderosis has also been observed in apparently primary amyloid disease (Green *et al.*, 1961).

While rectal biopsy is now well established as a valuable method for detecting generalized amyloid disease with a detection rate around 70 per cent, there can be little doubt that biopsy of the proximal small

Fig. 6.6 Transmission electron micrograph of lamina propria of small intestine in a case of intestinal amyloidosis. The cellular components are widely separated by dense bundles of fibrillar material with the ultrastructural characteristics of amyloid. Parts of several smooth muscle cells are seen here along with a small unmyelinated nerve.

intestine is equally effective. The possibility that amyloid may be present in an intestinal biopsy should always be entertained, regardless of the clinical circumstances. In the great majority of cases amyloid appears first and is most prominent in the submucosal blood vessels. Its presence should be suspected if the normal cellular structure of the vessel wall is replaced by a structureless and faintly eosinophilic material (Fig. 4.33). It is claimed that in the more common secondary forms the intima is the site of initial deposition ('peri-reticulin' distribution) whereas in primary amyloidosis the adventitia is affected first ('peri-collagen' distribution; Sohar *et al.*, 1967). In most instances, it is difficult to make this distinction histologically since the entire thickness of the vessel wall is replaced (Fig. 4.33). The histological staining methods used to confirm the presence of amyloid are outlined else-

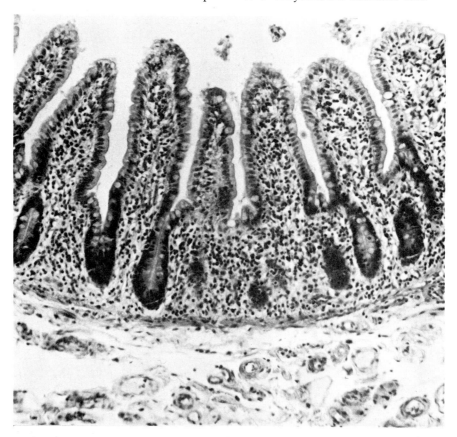

Fig. 6.7 Amyloidosis. The submucosal vessels are diffusely affected by amyloid deposition, and the overlying ileal mucosa shows partial villous atrophy. From a case of rheumatoid arthritis. HE × 180.

where; usually a section stained by Congo red or Sirius red and viewed under the polarizing microscope is sufficient for routine diagnostic purposes (Section 2.4). In cases of doubt, however, confirmation of the presence of amyloid can be obtained by demonstrating the characteristic fibrillary structure under the electron microscope (Fig. 6.6). In severe cases of intestinal amyloidosis the blood vessels of the lamina propria are involved (Fig. 4.33), and occasionally there is deposition of amyloid between muscle bundles in the lamina muscularis mucosae and beneath the epithelial basement membrane. Several intestinal lesions such as ulceration and ischaemic damage have been reported in association with amyloidosis and have usually been attributed to the occlusion of vascular lumina by amyloid deposition. Villous atrophy of crypt hyperplastic type (Section 4.2.1) has also been personally observed in resected segments of the small bowel affected by amyloid disease (Fig. 6.7). The extent to which amyloid deposition can be incriminated in the causation of these intestinal lesions is, however, debatable since intestinal biopsy studies have usually shown that the villous pattern is normal in amyloidosis even when malabsorption is suspected clinically (Green *et al.*, 1961).

References

Akbarian, M. and Fenton, J. (1964), Perforation of small bowel in amyloidosis. *Arch. intern. Med.*, **114**, 815–821.

Arapakis, G. and Tribe, C.P. (1963), Amyloidosis in rheumatoid arthritis. *Ann. rheum. Dis.*, **22**, 256–262.

Bero, G. L. (1957), Amyloidosis: its clinical and pathologic manifestations with a report of 12 cases. *Ann. intern. Med.*, **46**, 931–953.

Chears, W. C. Jr. and Ashworth, C. T. (1961), Electron microscopic study of the intestinal mucosa in Whipple's disease. *Gastroenterology*, **41**, 129–138.

Dobbins, W. O. (1966), Abetalipoproteinaemia. *Gastroenterology*, **50**, 195–210.

Farnan, P. (1965), In *The Small Intestine. A symposium of the 5th Congress of the International Academy of Pathology*. (Ed. Thackray, A. C. and Avery Jones, F.). Blackwell, Oxford.

Golden, R. (1954), Amyloidosis of the small intestine. *Am. J. Roentg.*, **72**, 401–408.

Green, P. A., Higgins, J. A., Brown, A. L., Hoffman, H. N. and Sommerville, R. L. (1961), Amyloidosis: appraisal of intubation biopsy of small intestine in diagnosis. *Gastronenterology*, **41**, 452–456.

Hourihane, D.O'B. (1966), The pathology of malabsorptive states. In *Recent Advances in Pathology* (Ed. Harrison, C. V.), 8th Edition. J. A. Churchill, London.

Kayden, H. J. (1972), Abetalipoproteinaemia. *A. Rev. Med.*, **23**, 285–296.

Lamy, M., Frezal, J., Polonouski, J., Druez, G. and Rey, J. (1963), Congenital absence of betalipoproteins. *Paediatrics*, **31**, 277–289.

Lee, F. D. (1966), Submucosal lipophages in diverticula of the small intestine. *J. Path. Bact.*, **92**, 29–34.

Lee, F. D., El-Ghobarey, A. F., Buchanan, W. W. and Browne, M. K. (1978), Rheumatoid arthritis, amyloidosis, intestinal ulceration, refractory iron deficiency anaemia and intestinal haemosiderosis: a new clinical syndrome? *Revue int. Rheumatol.*, **7**, 121–124.

Mistilis, S. P., Skyring, A. P. and Stephen D. D. (1965), Intestinal lymphangiectasia. Mechanism of enteric loss of plasma protein and fat. *Lancet*, **1**, 77–79.

Morningstar, W. A. (1975), Whipple's disease. An example of the value of the electron microscope in diagnosis, follow-up and correlation of a pathologic process. *Human Path.*, **6**, 443–454.

Pittman, F. E., Smith, W. T., Mizrahi, A., Blanc, W. A. and Pittman, J. C. (1966), Clinical histochemical and electron microscopic study of colonic histiocytosis. *Gut*, **7**, 458–467.

Pruzanski, W., Warren, R., Goldie, J. and Katz, A. (1973), Malabsorption syndrome with infiltration of the intestinal wall by extracellular monoclonal macroglobulin. *Am. J. Med.*, **54**, 811–818.

Rubin, C. E. and Dobbins, W. O. (1965), Peroral biopsy of the small intestine. A review of its diagnostic usefulness. *Gastroenterology*, **49**, 676–697.

Salt, H. B., Wolff, O. H., Lloyd, J. K., Fosbrooke, A. S., Cameron, A. H. and Hubble, D. V. (1960), On having no betalipoprotein. A syndrome comprising abetalipoproteinaemia, acanthocytosis and steatorrhoea. *Lancet*, **2**, 325–329.

Shilken, K. B., Zerman, B. J. and Blackwell, J. B. (1968), Lymphangiectatic cysts of the small bowel. *J. Path. Bact.*, **96**, 353–358.

Sohar, E., Merker, H. J., Missmahl, H. P., Fagni, J. and Heller, H. (1967), Electron microscope observations on peri-reticulin and peri-collagen amyloidosis in rectal biopsies. *J. Path. Bact.*, **94**, 89–93.

Strober, W., Wochner, R. D., Carbone, P. P. and Waldmann, T. A. (1967), Intestinal lymphangiectasia: a protein-losing enteropathy with hypogammaglobulinaemia, lymphocytopenia and impaired homograft rejection. *J. clin. Invest.*, **46**, 1643–1656.

Waldmann, T. A. (1966), Protein-losing enteropathy. *Gastroenterology*, **50**, 422–443.

Whipple, G. H. (1907), A hitherto undescribed disease characterized anatomically by deposits of fat and fatty acids in the intestinal and mesenteric lymphatic tissues. *Bull. Johns Hopkins. Hosp.*, **18**, 382–391.

Yardley, J. H. and Hendrix, R. T. (1961), Combined electron and light microscopy in Whipple's disease. *Bull. Johns Hopkins Hosp.*, **109**, 80–98.

7 Abnormalities in other disease states

7.1 Crohn's Disease

7.1.1 General features

This chronic inflammatory disorder of unknown aetiology can affect any part of the alimentary tract from the oral cavity to the anus. The small intestine, and in particular the most distal part of the ileum, is still, however, the site most commonly involved. While recent histological studies suggest that Crohn's disease may produce more diffuse inflammatory changes than was previously thought (Dunne *et al.*, 1977), the lesions visible to the naked eye are characteristically patchy or 'discontinuous' in distribution, and unpredictable with regard to their extent. This last feature accounts for the notorious propensity of the disease to recur after surgical resections. The irregularity in the distribution of the lesions makes it unlikely that random intestinal biopsy would be of much value in the diagnosis of Crohn's disease, with the exception of unusual cases in which there is widespread involvement of the upper small bowel (see Fig. 4.32). Even then, a biopsy consisting mainly of mucosa seldom reveals diagnostic lesions; mucosal changes are much more likely to be non-specific and secondary to distinctive alterations taking place at a deeper level in the intestinal wall.

The gross thickening of the intestine characteristic of the disease is due mainly to chronic inflammatory reaction and oedema which not only involve the entire thickness of the bowel wall but extend into the related mesentery and lymph nodes. The chronic inflammatory reaction has two components which may be regarded as typical. The first is focal lymphocytic infiltration, found in all cases and at all stages in the disease. Lymphoid aggregates, sometimes showing germinal centres, are most conspicuous in the submucosa although often seen in the serosal coat and mesentery. In some cases they invaginate dilated lymphatic channels (Fig. 7.1).

The sarcoid reaction or 'giant-cell system' (Section 4.1.3) is the other feature typical and probably more characteristic of Crohn's disease although it can be found only in about two-thirds of cases. While this change may be seen in all layers of the bowel wall, and in the mesenteric lymph nodes, it is always most easily found in the submucosa and at the seroso-muscular junction. The sarcoid follicles are indistinguishable from those of non-caseating tuberculosis or sarcoidosis, and the giant cells may contain a variety of inclusions, including conchoid Schaumann bodies. The sarcoid reaction may first become evident within lymphoid aggregates (Hadfield, 1939). In about 40 per cent of cases, however, they arise close to or actually within lymphatic channels (see Warren and Sommers, 1948; Fig. 7.2) and solitary giant cells are sometimes seen in lymphatics. Sclerosis and hyalinization of these peri-lymphatic sarcoid follicles is occasionally demonstrable (Fig. 7.3). Very rarely, the sarcoid reaction involves blood vessels, and may be associated with fibrinoid necrosis of arterial walls.

Diffuse submucosal inflammatory infiltration may also be found in addition to these local lesions; plasma cells, eosinophils and lymphocytes predominate, but histiocytes and occasional mast cells are also seen. This diffuse type of inflammation is usually associated with granulation tissue formation particularly in relation to ulcers and fissures (v.i.). Oedema is an outstanding feature of the disease process, especially in the earlier phases, and is invariably associated with engorgement of lymphatic channels. Always most conspicuous in the submucosa, oedema gives way to fibrosis and even fat deposition in the later phases of the disease. The formation of fissures extending through the submucosa and muscularis propria is a common and important phenomenon, and accounts for the occurrence of serosal or peri-intestinal abscesses and the development of fistulae extending into adjacent hollow viscera or through the skin of the abdominal wall. Fissure tracks are lined by granulation tissue with a surface layer of neutrophils: giant cells, usually of foreign-body type, are often seen close to the surface and are to be distinguished from true sarcoid follicles. Other features of interest include focal hypertrophy of the lamina muscularis mucosae (Van Patter et al., 1954), hypertrophy of the muscularis propria, and undue prominence of the neural compo-

---

Fig. 7.1 Crohn's disease. Focal lymphocytic infiltration with germinal centre formation lying in close relationship to a submucosal lymphatic channel. A sarcoid reaction is also developing towards the left-hand side of the lymphoid aggregate. HE × 130.

Fig. 7.2 Crohn's disease. A sarcoid reaction is developing within a subserosal lymphatic channel. HE × 160.

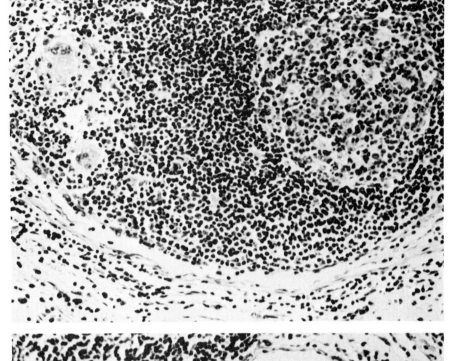

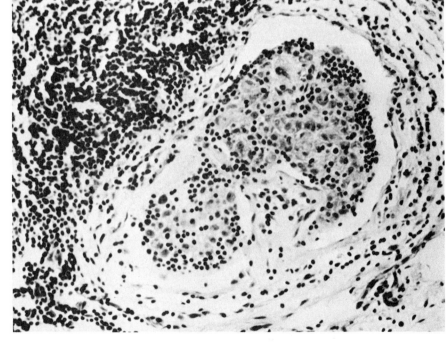

nents of the submucosal and myenteric plexuses ('neuromatous' change; Rappaport *et al.*, 1951). Apart from rare involvement by the sarcoid reaction (see above) endarteritis obliterans is the only notable change in blood vessels.

Mucosal changes. While the diagnosis of Crohn's disease usually rests upon histological changes in the deeper layers of the intestinal wall, the characteristic sarcoid reaction is found in the mucosa in about 15 per cent of cases and may be found at some distance from the obvious macroscopic lesions. It is rare however for a mucosal sarcoid follicle to be detected by jejunal biopsy, and even when a biopsy includes sub-mucosal tissue it is unusual for a positive diagnosis to be possible. The sarcoid reaction is much more often seen in colonic mucosal biopsies. It is the authors' impression that colonic Crohn's disease more often remains confined to the mucosa and submucosa than is the case in classical ileal Crohn's disease. The success rate in biopsy diagnosis is greater in the colon because colonic biopsies can usually be taken from visually identified abnormal areas.

Much more often the mucosal changes in the small intestine are entirely non-specific in nature. Random jejunal biopsy studies in patients with Crohn's disease have, for example, shown that in some patients there may be diffuse or extensive villous atrophy usually of mild or partial degree (Shiner and Drury, 1963). The most serious changes, which inevitably culminate in frank ulceration, are, however, strikingly co-terminous with the macroscopic transmural lesions, and correspond in broad terms to the localized hypertrophic villous pattern (Section 4.2.2). Initially, the villi become grossly distended by conges-tion, oedema, lymphangiectasis and leucocytic infiltration which, while essentially non-specific, is sometimes characterized by intense accumulation of small lymphocytes (Fig. 4.32). At a later phase, fib-rosis and hyalinization of the villous lamina propria become conspicu-ous (Fig. 4.20). Crypt abscess formation often develops in severe cases, and this, together with the fusion of markedly inflamed hypertrophic villi ('pseudo-atrophy', Section 4.2.2, Fig. 4.44) almost always heralds the onset of ulceration. Sometimes there is a brief transition to a true atrophic pattern (Section 4.2.1) prior to frank ulceration. Foci of villous atrophy may also be found at some distance from the transmural

Fig. 7.3 Crohn's disease. A sarcoid follicle undergoing sclerosis within a subserosal lymphatic channel. HE × 180.

Fig. 7.4 Crohn's disease. In this case there were diffuse lesions in the upper small bowel, and a random jejunal biopsy showed nonspecific mucosal inflammation together with a small focus of gastric metaplasia. Note the basally situated nuclei in the metaplastic glands. HE × 510.

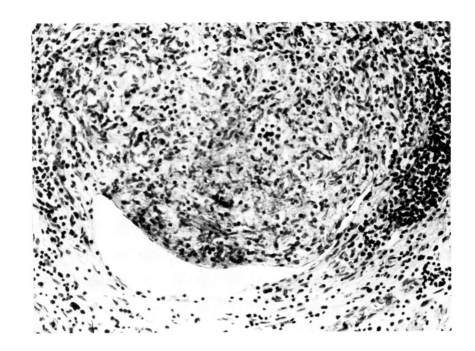

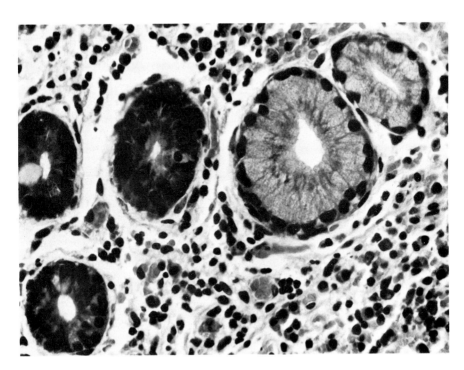

lesions and tend to develop at the tops of mucosal folds. This phenomenon may well account for the atrophic changes which have been reported in random jejunal biopsies in cases of Crohn's disease, and is probably due to intestinal obstruction with consequent stasis and abnormal luminal bacterial growth.

Gastric metaplasia is found in over two-thirds of cases of Crohn's disease (Liber, 1951; Lee, 1964), and is usually associated with ulceration (Fig. 4.17); sometimes, however, foci of metaplasia are seen at some distance from the ulcerative lesions. While metaplasia is by no means a specific change (Section 4.1.2) its presence in a random jejunal biopsy should always raise the suspicion of Crohn's disease (Fig. 7.4).

Morson (1972) has drawn attention to the occurrence of tiny 'aphthoid ulcers' in the apparently normal mucosa in cases of Crohn's disease, suggesting that these small foci, usually centred on small lymphoid follicles, might form the basis for the eventual development of further 'skip' lesions. The scanning microscope shows these lesions with particular clarity (Fig. 7.5), demonstrating a distinctive orderly petal-like arrangement of the surrounding villi. Epithelial cell 'bridging' of adjacent villi has also been reported on the basis of this study (Rickert and Carter, 1977).

7.1.2 Endoscopic biopsy in Crohn's disease

While it is seldom possible to detect the lesions of Crohn's disease in the small bowel by endoscopic means, the disease has occasionally been observed in the duodenum or in the terminal ileum (during endoscopy) and biopsies taken under direct vision.

As mentioned above 'granulomatous' lesions are seen in the small bowel mucosa in only a minority of cases, and have not been personally found in endoscopic mucosal biopsies. Nevertheless, a diagnosis of Crohn's disease can still be suspected from the presence of certain characteristic mucosal changes. Focal inflammatory reaction in the lamina propria is especially useful diagnostically although it must be clearly distinguished from normal lymphoid follicles. This inflamma-

Fig. 7.5 Dissecting micrograph (a) and scanning electron micrograph (b) of small intestinal mucosa in a case of Crohn's disease. The small focus of ulceration which is arrowed in (a) can be clearly seen in (b). These focal lesions are thought to represent the earliest stage of the mucosal injury in Crohn's disease. A zone of congestion is seen around the ulcer in the dissecting micrograph, while the scanning micrograph shows particularly clearly the petal-like arrangement of the villi and suggests some degree of villous fusion. Micrographs by courtesy of Dr R. R. Rickert. (Rickert and Carter, 1977.)

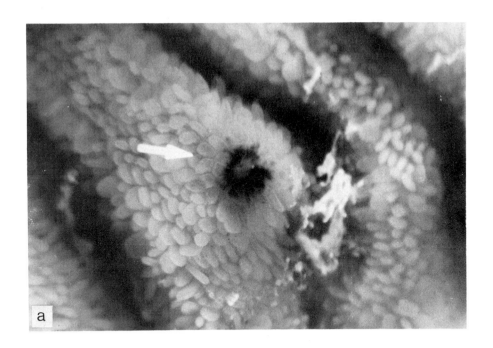

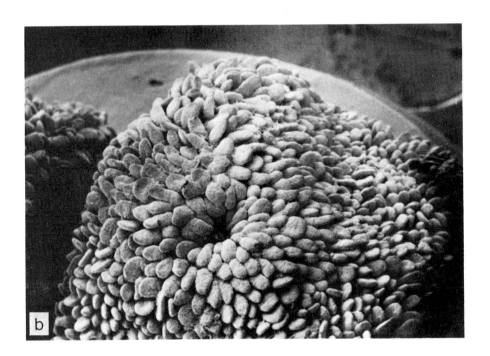

tory infiltrate often shows a high proportion of small lymphocytes, and commonly there is associated lymphatic dilatation. The presence of gastric metaplasia, while by no means specific, is nevertheless strongly suggestive of Crohn's disease. The focal aphthoid ulcers already referred to may also be diagnostically useful.

7.1.3. The pathogenesis of the intestinal lesions

The aetiology of Crohn's disease is still unknown. Recent studies including electron microscopy, suggest that a transmissible agent is involved (Aronson *et al.*, 1974, Cave *et al.*, 1975; Riemann, 1977), and the close similarity of the lesions to those of tuberculosis (see below) would support this possibility. All the evidence suggests that the initial histological event is the appearance of a sarcoid reaction at any point between the mucosa and the regional mesenteric lymph nodes, and even beyond. The causation of the subsequent histological changes is much less certain, although for the most part they can be attributed to widespread lymphatic obstruction and oedema of the bowel wall. The observation that sarcoid follicles quite often arise in or around lymphatics, and tend to become sclerosed and hyalinized, provides a possible explanation for this lymphatic disturbance. It is tempting to suppose that Crohn's disease is due to a transmissible agent, which in susceptible individuals gains access to the intestinal lymphatics, there elicits a chronic inflammatory response and as a result produces extensive lymphatic occlusion. Apart from the uncommon intramucosal sarcoid follicles, the mucosal changes mainly result either from oedema with secondary infection or from the effects of chronic intestinal obstruction and stasis (Section 4.2.2).

7.1.4 Differential diagnosis

As mentioned in Section 4.1.3, it is rare for a sarcoid reaction in the intestinal wall to be caused by any condition other than Crohn's disease. The possibility of tuberculosis however must always be seriously considered, since the histological features can be identical in every respect. Only the unequivocal presence of caseation in the sarcoid follicles and of tubercle bacilli enable tuberculosis to be distinguished with certainty from Crohn's disease. Even although tuberculosis of the intestinal tract is becoming increasingly uncommon in developed countries it is still unwise to omit the use of the Ziehl-Neelsen stain in supposed cases of Crohn's disease. Culture or guinea pig inoculation of fresh unfixed tissue from the intestinal lesions removed at operation has much to commend it.

7.2 Radiation enteritis

Damage to the small intestine by ionizing radiation usually arises as a complication after the treatment of pelvic or intra-abdominal cancer, the extent and severity being dependent upon the dosage of irradiation and the method by which it is given. Intestinal obstruction, sometimes associated with perforation and fistula formation, is the most common clinical disturbance and tends to be associated with localized damage as may occur, for example, when a loop of small bowel is accidentally included in the field of irradiation for carcinoma of the cervix uteri. Malabsorption, also a well-recognized effect, tends to develop at two distinct phases in relationship to a course of irradiation. First, diarrhoea and malabsorption, usually of mild degree, may arise as an acute phenomenon during or immediately after a course of radiotherapy (Reeves et al., 1959); while this may persist or recur, it is usually transient, and is probably caused by damage to the epithelial stem cells (enteroblasts) with temporary impairment of enterocyte production. Secondly, and more commonly, malabsorption arises at a later phase, its onset being delayed for as much as 5 to 6 months after an episode of irradiation (Tankel et al., 1965). The cause is not entirely clear: mucosal damage does not appear to be of primary importance. In some respects, this delayed form of malabsorptive disturbance resembles that observed in the blind loop syndrome and is presumably related to intestinal stasis (Section 5.4). It is thus not without relevance that many of the late effects of irradiation are attributable to progressive vascular occlusion and ischaemic damage to the intestinal wall, which result in defective intestinal motility and chronic intestinal obstruction. Marked lipofuscinosis of the intestinal wall, probably due to protein-losing enteropathy, may also be observed. Lymphatic obstruction and fistula formation may contribute to the development of malabsorption.

Relatively little is known histologically in man about the intestinal changes taking place during the 'acute' phase of exposure to ionizing radiation. In the jejunum, varying degrees of villous collapse, leading ultimately to a completely 'flat' mucosa, have been reported, the changes being maximal about 11 days after irradiation. The appearances broadly correspond to the hypoplastic villous pattern (Section 4.2.3) and are presumably due to epithelial stem-cell (enteroblast) damage. The villous pattern may alter rapidly, presumably as a result of variations in enterocyte replacement (Carr and Toner, 1972; Anderson and Withers 1973); on the other hand, the pattern may remain static for as long as 6 months or more (Wiernik, 1966).

Mucosal alteration may thus form part of the histological picture observed in the later or delayed phase of radiation damage to the small intestine. More often, however, this phase is recognized by changes taking place in the deeper layers of the bowel wall and usually only found in surgical resections. These changes are as follows. There is oedema, most noticeable in the submucosa (Fig. 7.6) and becoming evident 3 – 6 months after irradiation; there is fibrosis and hyalinization of connective tissue, a much later change seldom seen before 15 months; there occurs vascular damage, usually manifested by hyalinization of arterial walls (Fig. 7.7) with intimal thickening, or dilatation of small blood vessels and lymphatics (telangiectasis), seen at about 9 – 10 months; and there are found atypical mesenchymal cells ('irradiation fibroblasts') of stellate shape, with abundant basophilic cytoplasm and large folded or irregular nuclei with prominent nucleoli. These cells may be present at an early phase and at all levels in the gut wall; they are often, however, most conspicuous at the bases of ulcers (Fig. 7.8). This cellular change, undoubtedly the most useful diagnostically, may still be visible as long as 12 years after irradiation.

The mucosal changes observed in relationship to the delayed phase are extremely variable. Occasionally, the appearances are those of severe crypt hypoplastic villous atrophy (Fig. 4.47) which may be found as long as 9 months after irradiation. Presumably this change is caused by inadequate recovery from enteroblast damage sustained during the acute phase, although it is possible that mucosal ischaemia developing due to vascular change may be a contributory factor. Sometimes the mucosal features more closely resemble crypt hyperplastic partial villous atrophy (Fig. 7.6), especially during the period 3–4 months after irradiation. This alteration probably represents a phase of recovery from enteroblast damage, and it is notable that unlike the atrophic villous pattern observed in other disease states (Section 4.2.1) the enterocytes at the villous extremity appear normal. Paneth cells and argentaffin cells may also be unusually conspicuous; it seems that these cells are relatively resistant to radiation damage (Friedman, 1945). Finally, the mucosal changes may be those of the localized hypertrophic villous pattern (Section 4.2.2) especially in those cases in which intestinal obstruction has been the presenting clinical disturbance. This alteration is not, of course, directly related to irradiation damage, although it adds emphasis to the point that any form of intestinal damage may be exploited by potentially pathogenic micro-organisms in the intestinal lumen.

Fig. 7.6 Radiation enteritis. The mucosa in this case presents an appearance similar to crypt hyperplastic partial villous atrophy. Note also the striking degree of submucosal oedema. HE × 100.

Fig. 7.7 Radiation enteritis. Submucosal arteries showing marked narrowing and hyalinization. HE × 225.

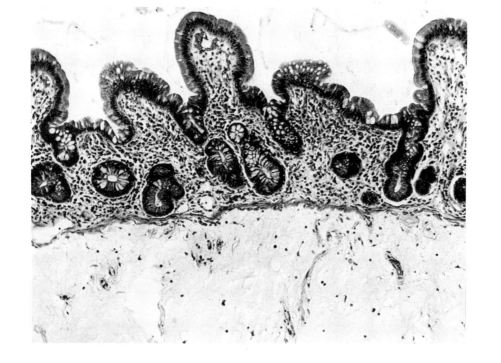

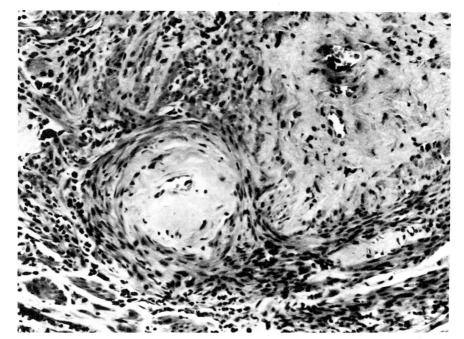

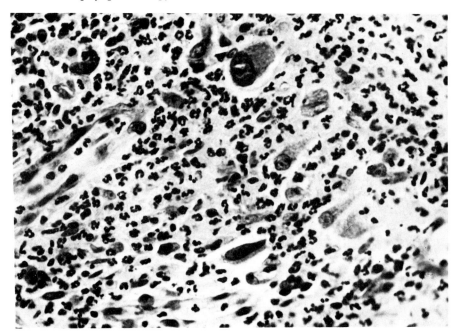

Fig. 7.8 Radiation enteritis. Atypical mesenchymal cells ('irradiation fibro-blasts') in the jejunal submucosa. HE × 580.

7.3 Eosinophilic enteritis

The eosinophil polymorph is an ubiquitous cell in the mucosa of the gastro-intestinal tract both under normal conditions and in most types of inflammatory reaction. Apart from occasional cases of giardiasis (Section 7.7) and helminthic infection (Section 7.8), however, it is unusual for the eosinophil to be the predominant cell in inflammatory states. Perhaps the most notable example in adults is the condition known as eosinophilic gastro-enteritis. The causation of this disease is still uncertain. While infestation with the herring parasite *Eustoma rotundatum* has been incriminated in some instances (Kuipers *et al.*, 1960), it seems more probable that hypersensitivity to food allergens is responsible (see Leinbach and Rubin, 1970; Greenberger and Gryboski, 1973); a peripheral blood eosinophilia is commonly observed, and in some patients there is a history of atopic allergy. The clinical symptoms appear to be related to the nature of the pathological changes in the stomach or small bowel. With predominant involvement of the intestinal mucosa, malabsorptive disturbance or protein-losing enteropathy are the principal features. When the deeper layers of the gastro-intestinal tract are affected the symptoms are mainly obstructive: and, while the pylorus is the site most often involved, the small intestine may on occasion be implicated (see Greenberger and Gryboski, 1973). As might be expected, intestinal biopsy is more likely to be of diagnostic value in the mucosal form.

In histological terms, for reasons yet to be elucidated, the disease is often patchy whether the mucosa or the deeper parts of the intestinal wall are primarily affected. In the mucosal form, the outstanding histological feature is infiltration of the lamina propria by eosinophils, which may also be seen on occasion within the epithelial surface (Fig. 7.9). This cellular reaction may have little effect on villous architecture apart from slight villous swelling, but foci of partial or even subtotal villous atrophy may develop (Fig. 7.10). Degenerative change may be seen in the enterocytes of the villous extremity, and in severe cases neutrophil emigration through the epithelium becomes apparent, followed in a minority of cases by superficial ulceration. Some degree of submucosal oedema may be found in association with these mucosal lesions. In the 'obstructive' form of the disease, however, this is the predominant feature and the submucosa may measure more than 5 mm in thickness. The eosinophilic infiltration is mainly submucosal, although it may also extend into the muscularis propria or serosa: mast cells may accompany the eosinophils. Some submucosal fibrinous exudation may be present, tending to be most pronounced in the adventitia of small blood vessels, giving the impression of vasculitis. The overlying mucosa seldom shows any significant eosinophilia in the 'obstructive' form, but foci of partial or subtotal villous atrophy have been observed (Fig. 4.36).

The histological changes usually found in the mucosal form of eosinophilic enteritis are virtually indistinguishable from those of the childhood condition allergic gastro-enteropathy, which appears to be a hypersensitivity reaction to milk products, and is also associated clinically with malabsorption and protein-losing enteropathy (Waldmann et al., 1967). The obstructive form, when it arises in the small intestine, may be mistaken (especially at the macroscopic level) for Crohn's disease, although the histological absence of lymphoid aggregates and sarcoid follicles and the predominance of eosinophils in the inflammatory reaction should enable the conditions to be easily distinguished.

7.4 Ischaemic disease

Ischaemia of the intestinal wall can be produced by a number of different mechanisms. The extent and severity of the resulting damage are subject to considerable variation and are largely dependent upon the causative factors involved. In strangulation, as takes place for example within a hernial sac, damage is limited to the obstructed loop and its severity is simply related to the duration of vascular stasis. Following occlusion of the major mesenteric blood vessels, the severity of haemorrhagic infarction is also related to the duration of ischaemia, but the extent is dependent upon the efficacy of the collateral circulation. Massive infarction only takes place when a major vessel such as the superior mesenteric artery is completely occluded, but on rare occasions this event may be preceded by episodes of focal ischaemic damage with perforation (Marrash et al., 1962). Partial occlusion of the major mesenteric arteries may also be the basis of the 'abdominal angina' syndrome, characterized by post-prandial pain and occasionally by malabsorption (Mandell, 1957). It is doubtful, however, if this syndrome is accompanied by pathological change in the intestinal wall. Inflammatory disease of the mesenteric arterial system, most often due to polyarteritis nodosa, systemic lupus erythematosus or rheumatoid arthritis, may produce either focal or extensive confluent ischaemic damage to the small bowel. It is worth re-emphasizing that some of the pathological changes caused by ionizing radiation may also be fundamentally ischaemic in nature (Section 7.2). Impaired perfusion of the intestinal vasculature as a result of cardiac failure, shock or severe infection may also produce varying degrees of ischaemic damage dependent upon the duration of perfusion failure. In such cases occlusive disease of the major mesenteric arteries may also be a contributory factor and the lesions tend to arise in 'watershed' areas such as the splenic flexure ('ischaemic colitis'; see Marston et al., 1966). The small intestine, however, may also be affected by perfusion failure, resulting in ischaemic enterocolitis.

While the mucosa is the first part of the intestinal wall to show morphological change as a result of ischaemia, intestinal biopsy is only rarely of clinical value in the diagnosis of ischaemic disease of the small intestine. Nevertheless, it is important that ischaemic damage should be recognized histologically. The description that follows is based mainly upon histological studies of surgically resected specimens of small bowel.

Certain histological mucosal changes characterize the earliest recognizable phase of ischaemic damage. Swelling of the lamina propria due to oedema, with or without haemorrhage or vascular dilatation, is

---

Fig. 7.9 Eosinophilic enteritis (mucosal form). Eosinophils are prominent in the lamina propria and within the epithelial surface. HE × 820.

Fig. 7.10 Eosinophilic enteritis (mucosal form). There is patchy crypt hyperplastic villous atrophy. HE × 180.

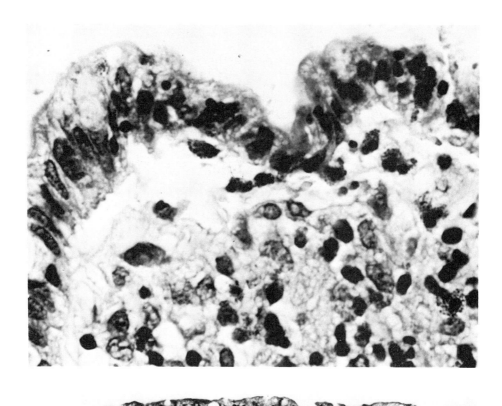
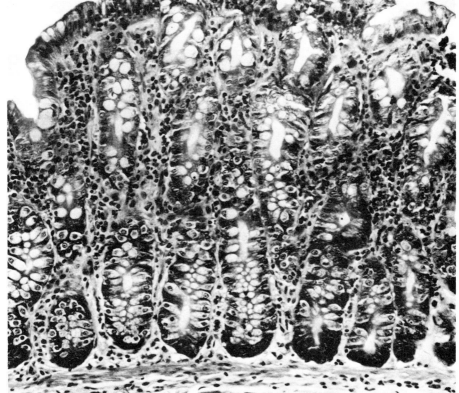

invariable and may lead to a measurable increase in villous width. Submucosal oedema may also be prominent. Emigration of neutrophils into the lamina propria and subsequently into the epithelium at the villous extremity (Fig. 4.21) is a typical finding and perhaps the most useful diagnostically. A mild crypt hypoplastic villous atrophy may also be present at an early phase (Fig. 7.11). Later, epithelial damage becomes evident, first at the villous extremity and especially at the summits of mucosal folds. Adhesions or 'synechiae' may develop between epithelial cells of adjacent villi, and may lead to crypt dilatation (Fig. 7.12). Ultimately, the epithelial cells of the villous surface and crypts become markedly attenuated, and the crypts appear atrophic (Fig. 7.13). Presumably these epithelial changes are largely due to a cessation of epithelial replacement, and certainly they herald the onset of frank ulceration which initially begins at the villous extremity. Fibrin thrombi do not usually appear in the capillaries of the lamina propria until this late phase has been reached. The more advanced stages of ischaemic damage in which there is massive necrosis of the mucosa and possibly of the deeper layers of the bowel wall are readily recognized histologically and do not require further discussion. Only in the case of the arteritic disturbances mentioned above, however, is it ever possible to be certain as to the cause of an ischaemic disturbance on histological grounds alone.

The neutrophil emigration into the villous epithelium characterizing the early phase of ischaemia is simply a consequence of epithelial damage, the same phenomenon being seen in the vicinity of almost any ulcerative lesion in the intestinal tract. In inflammatory or neoplastic states, however, it is usually associated with the localized hypertrophic villous pattern with or without pseudo-atrophic flattening of the villous architecture (Section 4.2.2), and there is usually a pronounced non-specific inflammatory response in the lamina propria (Fig. 4.44). This is in contrast to ischaemic damage in which such inflammatory change is minimal and there is commonly crypt hypoplastic villous atrophy. It should be mentioned, however, that following recovery from an ischaemic episode with ulceration, secondary bacterial infection may produce striking inflammatory change – both acute and chronic – in the ulcer base and surrounding tissues: indeed in more chronic cases the appearances may resemble Crohn's disease (Hawkins, 1957). In such instances the demonstration of widespread

Fig. 7.11 Ischaemic enteritis. An early lesion showing mild crypt hypoplastic villous atrophy. HE × 180.
Fig. 7.12 Ischaemic enteritis. In this case, mild hypoplastic villous atrophy is associated with foci of crypt dilatation. HE × 160.

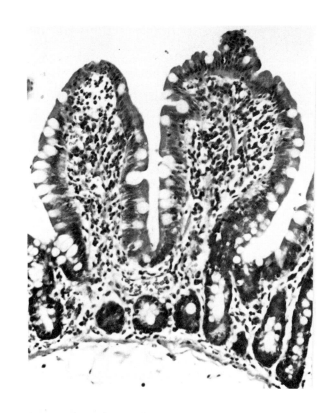

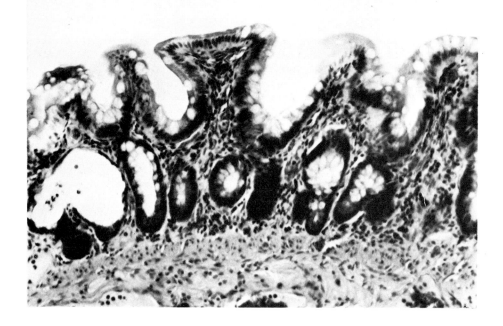

haemosiderin deposition in the intestinal wall may be a useful indication of previous ischaemic damage with haemorrhage (Price and
Morson, 1975).

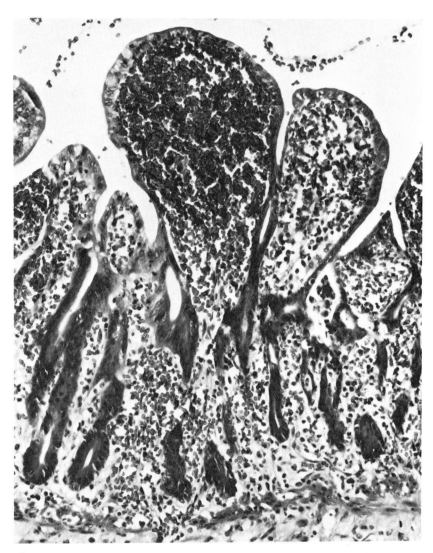

Fig. 7.13 Ischaemic enteritis. There is attenuation of the villous epithelium and
the crypts appear atrophic. Haemorrhage into the lamina propria is also a
notable feature. HE × 235.

7.5 Virus infections

The clinical picture of acute gastro-enteritis is commonly seen in practice. It is, however, rarely the subject of detailed hospital investigation and biopsy, since it is a short and generally self-limiting illness, the characteristic symptoms of nausea, vomiting and diarrhoea, with or without slight fever, usually passing off within a few days. In infants and children however, particularly when they are debilitated or malnourished, the metabolic disturbance of this illness may prove fatal. Acute gastroenteritis is, therefore, an important cause of morbidity and mortality among children in the poorer countries of the world. It is possible, too, that such an illness may act as a trigger for a more prolonged episode of intestinal malfunction, perhaps by unmasking an underlying defect such as mild gluten sensitivity. For these reasons the topic is worthy of attention.

Acute gastro-enteritis, whether sporadic or epidemic, is often clearly transmissible, and in many cases cannot be attributed to any known bacterial, toxic or parasitic cause. A viral cause had thus long been suspected, both on clinical and experimental grounds. For many years, however, culture studies were unsuccesful and the extent to which viruses were actually involved in this clinical syndrome, and the identity of these viruses, remained uncertain.

Electron microscopy has been of importance in the investigation of this problem (Almeida, 1975; Schreiber *et al.*, 1977). Bishop *et al.* (1973) were the first to demonstrate the occurrence of virus-like particles within damaged intestinal epithelial cells in infantile gastro-enteritis (Fig. 7.14a). They subsequently confirmed that similar-sized particles could be detected by the direct examination of negatively stained faecal samples. The virus particles, 65 nm in diameter when their outer shells are retained, resemble the Reovirus groups. The term Rotavirus is the most widely accepted at the present time to identify this infection (Fig. 7.14b). This is the major cause of infantile transmissible non-bacterial gastro-enteritis in many countries around the world.

A second virus class has been implicated in other outbreaks, in particular the much studied Norwalk epidemic. The agent in this case is 27 nm in diameter, and is classified as a parvovirus. It is seen only when the faecal particles have been agglutinated by precipitation with immune serum and concentrated by subsequent centrifugation. This technique, known as immune electron microscopy, is of great value in such studies, but does not permit clear visualization of virus morphology, since the particles are coated with antibody.

Several other viruses have been identified in association with clinical outbreaks of gastro-enteritis, although asymptomatic excretion may

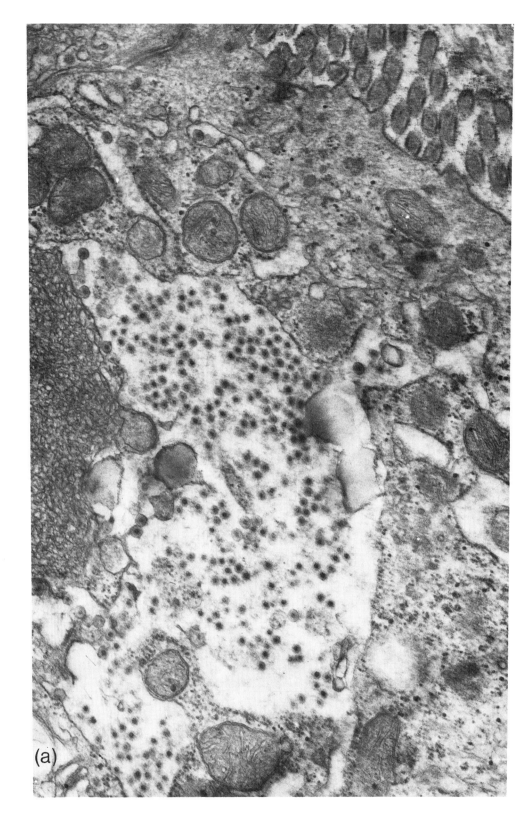

(a)

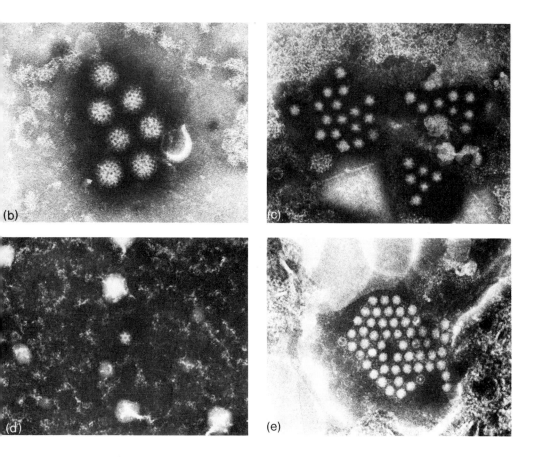

Fig. 7.14(a) Transmission electron micrograph of small intestinal biopsy from an infant with rotavirus infection. Note the presence of virus particles within distended cytoplasmic spaces, apparently continuous with the rough endoplasmic reticulum. This micrograph, by courtesy of Dr R. F. Bishop, provided the first documentary evidence of virus infection in association with non-bacterial gastroenteritis in children. (Bishop *et al.*, 1973)

(b)–(e) Negatively stained viruses observed in faeces from infants with non-bacterial enteritis. (b) Rotavirus. This is the most frequently observed faecal virus. It is 65–70 nm in diameter, with a structure superficially similar to the reoviruses. (c) Astrovirus. This virus is 28 nm in diameter with a proportion of virions showing a 5- or 6-pointed surface star. (d) Calicivirus. This is 33 nm in diameter with cup-shaped surface hollows. The clear-cut 6-pointed star with a central hole and the more feathery edge, distinguish this from the astrovirus. (e) 'Small round viruses'. Such particles are variable in size and detailed appearance. Particles of this type may include bacteriophages. Micrographs by courtesy of Dr A. R. Madeley.

also occur. The astrovirus is a 28 nm smooth-surfaced virus, which frequently has a five- or six-pointed star configuration. The calcivirus is 29 nm in diameter, with a feathery outside edge and a central hole within a Star of David configuration. Coronaviruses, irregular in shape with club-like projections, have been implicated in some cases. In addition to the above, various other small round objects, probably viral, can be detected in stools by direct electron microscopy (Fig. 7.14b). While many of these may simply be bacteriophages, the possible involvement of some of them in clinical disease cannot be excluded. Many of the virus classes described above are already known to be the cause of similar illnesses in neonatal animals of various species.

Biopsy studies of viral gastro-enteritis have shown the occurrence of various morphological abnormalities (Agus *et al.*, 1973; Schreiber *et al.*, 1977). There is shortening of the villi, hyperplasia of the crypts and infiltration of the lamina propria with polymorphs and mononuclears. Cuboidalisation and vacuolation of the surface cells are accompanied by ultrastructural evidence of damage to the endoplasmic reticulum, mitochondria and microvilli, and by widening of intercellular spaces and increased numbers of lysosomes. These changes, however, are non-specific. If seen in a biopsy unsupported by a clear clinical history, they would be indistinguishable from the similar non-specific changes reported in many other conditions. Studies of the gastric mucosa have shown no evidence of damage: the vomiting is probably all due to the intestinal abnormality and its constitutional consequences.

In the three of Bishop's cases which were re-examined by biopsy four to eight weeks after the acute illness, entirely normal appearances were found both by histology and by ultrastructure. It remains possible, however that in some cases a viral infection can lead to more persistent abnormalities of the intestinal mucosa, and may trigger off, or unmask, a previously latent tendency to malabsorption. On the other hand, there are occasional reported cases of 'coeliac disease', with subsequent total 'remission' even after discontinuing a gluten-free diet. Cases such as this might simply represent a transient post-viral malabsoption, which has remitted simultaneously with the initiation of a gluten-free diet, although not because of that therapy. Thus the possibility of viral disease must be kept in mind in the interpretation of minor biopsy abnormalities, and the full clinical history must always be scrutinized, to avoid possible errors of diagnosis.

The potential of direct electron microscopy in acute disease should also be kept in mind, since much detailed epidemiological work remains to be done in the acute gastroenteritis syndrome. Since the

viruses are resistant to culture the only available means of identification is electron microscopy. Moreover this technique has the advantage of permitting the detection of any virus present in sufficient
concentration in the faecal sample, irrespective of the availability of a
specific antiserum for immunological identification.

7.6 Other infective forms of enteritis

Apart from the infantile forms of gastro-enteritis described above,
intestinal biopsy is only rarely of value in the diagnosis of bacterial,
viral or fungal disease of the intestinal tract. During the enteric phase
of typhoid fever, distinctive lesions develop in the small bowel, but are
generally restricted to the solitary lymphoid follicles or lymphoid
aggregates of the mucosa, especially in the ileum. The leucocyte
response is lympho-plasmacytic in type and is typically accompanied
by cells of the mononuclear phagocyte system, which usually have
swollen eosinophilic cytoplasm often containing ingested nuclear
debris and red cells ('typhoid histiocytes'). Extensive areas of necrosis
develop in the affected lymphoid aggregates in severe cases. Neutrophil infiltration is only observed in the ulcerating surfaces of such
necrotic lesions. In personally studied autopsy cases, there has been
no evidence of a diffuse mucosal inflammatory lesion. Despite the
severe functional mucosal disturbance which characterizes cholera,
intestinal biopsy studies have generally failed to detect any mucosal
lesion (Gangarosa et al., 1960). Recent ultrastructural studies have,
however, demonstrated changes both in absorptive cells and 'undifferentiated' crypt cells as well as widening of interpithelial spaces in
the mid-villous zone (Asakura et al., 1974). These alterations have been
regarded as the morphological expression of accelerated fluid transport across the epithelial surface.

   In Britain, fungal disease such as candidosis is only seen as a rule in
immunosuppressed individuals. In other parts of the world, including
the U.S.A., histoplasmosis may affect the small intestine and produce
malabsorption in apparently normal individuals. The villi become
grossly distended as a result of infiltration by histiocytes which contain
the encapsulated organisms (Bank et al., 1965).

   In rare instances, viral diseases such as infectious mononucleosis or
measles have been shown to produce distinctive leucocytic alterations
in the lamina propria of the intestinal mucosa. In the latter case,
changes are more often found in the appendix than in the small bowel
and principally affect the lymphoid aggregates; the lymphoid fields
surrounding germinal centres may show pronounced 'immunoblastic'
activity associated with the characteristic multi-nucleated 'Warthin-

Finkeldey' cells (Fig. 4.25). Cytomegalovirus infection of the intestine is usually restricted to individuals with states of immunodeficiency, either congenital or acquired as a result of immunosuppressive agents. The lamina propria may contain numerous cells of presumptive histiocytic origin showing large intranuclear inclusions usually surrounded by a clear zone, the chromatin being condensed beneath the nuclear membrane; the cytoplasm may also be distended by viral inclusions. Other leucocytic components are sparse, and extensive villous atrophy may be a notable feature (Fig. 4.24).

7.7 Giardiasis

Colonization of the lumen of the small intestine by the flagellate protozoon parasite, *Giardia lamblia*, has been encountered in many parts of the world and, although especially common in the tropics, is by no means rare in Europe or North America. There now seems little doubt that this organism is capable of producing symptoms, especially diarrhoea; intestinal malabsorption has been reported in over 70 per cent of symptomatic patients (Wright, Tomkins and Ridley, 1977). It is also suspected that giardiasis is an important cause of malabsorption in immunologically deficient individuals (Ament and Rubin, 1972; Section 5.5). The diagnosis is usually made by examination of the stools for cysts, although the vegetative forms of the parasite can usually be readily recognized in intestinal biopsies stained by haemalum-eosin (Fig. 4.2). In suspected cases, however, the cytological examination of aspirated intestinal juice or mucus adherent to the surface of biopsies is recommended as the most reliable method for confirming the presence of parasites (Section 4.1.1).

The parasite is usually found on histology within the intestinal lumen or adherent to the epithelial surface (Fig. 4.2), although it is doubtful if parasites ever actually invade the epithelial surface. Minor villous abnormalities associated with an increase in leucocytic cells – especially eosinophils – have been reported, especially in tropically acquired cases with malabsorption (Wright *et al.*, 1977). Villous atrophy associated with giardiasis also undoubtedly occurs in immunodeficient individuals (Fig. 5.10) and may respond to appropriate therapy. In personally studied cases of giardiasis developing in immunologically normal individuals with malabsorption from the west of Scotland, however, the intestinal mucosa has usually been entirely normal both with regard to villous architecture and leucocytic infiltration. In occasional cases, the villous width is slightly increased due to a non-specific increase in leucocytes in the lamina propria, although eosinophils are not unduly prominent; the villous height may be at the

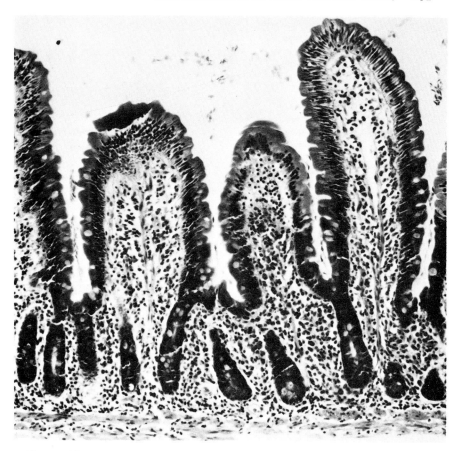

Fig. 7.15 Giardiasis. The villous height is at the lower limit of normal and there is a non-specific increase in leucocytic infiltration in the lamina propria. HE × 180.

lower limit of normal and the crypt : villus ratio in the 'high-normal' range (Fig. 7.15), but frank villous atrophy has not been observed. It thus seems improbable that disturbances in villous architecture are responsible for the malabsorption in giardiasis. More probably, heavy colonization with occlusion of the epithelial surfaces by parasites, or associated abnormal bacterial growth in the intestinal lumen are the cause.

7.8 Helminthic and other parasitic diseases

The lumen of the small intestine may harbour a large variety of metazoan parasites which are capable of producing severe intestinal disturbances and are responsible for extensive morbidity and even death especially in tropical or developing countries (Knight *et al.*, 1973). Of particular importance in this respect are the various forms of hookworm disease, such as that caused by the nematodes *Ankylostoma duodenale* and *Necator americanus* (Fig. 4.1). They produce their clinical effects mainly as a result of chronic blood loss, although they are also thought to be capable of causing intestinal malabsorption. The small intestine may also be affected in schistosomiasis (Halsted *et al.*, 1969). In many parts of the world infestation with another nematode *Strongyloides stercoralis*, while often symptomless, has also been reported as a cause of diarrhoea and malabsorption. In the Philippines, diarrhoea with severe malabsorption and protein-losing enteropathy has been attributed to the nematode *Capillaria philippinensis* (Whalen *et al.*, 1969; also *Lancet*, 1973). Parasites of this kind are rarely encountered in Europe or North America except in immigrants who have recently been resident in the tropics (Salem and Truelove, 1964). The sporozoan disease coccidiosis has also been reported to produce malabsorption with crypt hyperplastic villous atrophy, and can be detected by intestinal biopsy (Trier *et al.*, 1974). Severe intestinal disturbance caused by another coccidial disease crypto-sporidiosis has also been diagnosed by intestinal biopsy in an immunosuppressed individual (Meisel *et al.*, 1976; Nime *et al.*, 1976).

While the diagnosis of metazoan infestation is usually made by identification of the characteristic ova in the stools, the adult worms may on occasion be detected histologically in intestinal biopsies, especially in patients with heavy infestation. The organisms are normally found in the intestinal lumen and especially within the crypts of Lieberkühn (Fig. 4.1). Occasionally the organisms appear to be embedded within the lamina propria. While mucosal changes have been described in the upper small bowel in hookworm infestation (Sheehy *et al.*, 1962; Salem and Truelove, 1964), they are not consistently found and their significance is doubtful. In East Africa there is no relationship between jejunal mucosal morphology and the hookworm load (Cook *et al.*, 1969). Infestation with *Strongyloides stercoralis* has also been reported to produce duodenitis and jejunitis (Bras *et al.*, 1964) but here too there is overlap with similar changes often found in normal individuals resident in the tropics (Section 3.2). Similarly in capillariasis, it is doubtful if the parasite is capable of producing diffuse mucosal change. It is probable, however, that foci of crypt hyperplastic villous atrophy with increased leucocytic infiltration, and possible eosinophilia in the lamina propria, may be found at the sites of attachment of parasites to the epithelial surface.

References

Agus, S. G., Dolin, R., Wyatt, R. G., Tousimis, A. J. and Northrup, R. S. (1973), Acute infectious non-bacterial gastroenteritis: intestinal histopathology. *Ann. intern. Med.*, **79**, 18–25.

Almeida, J. D. (1975), Editorial: visualization of faecal viruses. *New. Engl. J. Med.*, **292**, 1403–1405.

Ament, M. and Rubin, C. E. (1972), Relation of giardiasis to abnormal intestinal structure and function in gastrointestinal immunodeficiency syndromes. *Gastroenterology*, **62**, 216–226.

Anderson, J. H. and Withers, R. H. (1973), Scanning electron microscope studies of irradiated rat intestinal mucosa. SEM/1973, 565–572. IITRI Chicago.

Aronson, M. D., Phillips, C. A. and Beeken, W. L. (1974), Isolation of a viral agent from intestinal tissue of patients with Crohn's disease and other intestinal disorders. *Gastroenterology*, **66**, 661. (Abstract)

Asakura, H., Tsuchiya, M., Watanabe, Y., Enomoto, Y., Morita, A., Morishita, A., Fukumi, H., Ohashi, M., Castro, A., and Uylanogc, C. (1974), Electron microscopic study on the jejunal mucosa in human cholera. *Gut*, **15**, 531–544.

Bank, S., Trey, C., Gaus, I., Marks, I. N. and Groll, A. (1965), Histoplasmosis of the small bowel with 'giant' intestinal villi and secondary protein-losing enteropathy. *Am. J. Med.*, **39**, 492–501.

Bishop, R. F., Davidson, G. P., Holmes, I. H. and Ruck, B. J. (1973), Virus particles in epithelial cells of duodenal mucosa from children with acute non-bacterial gastroenteritis. *Lancet*, **2**, 1281–1283.

Bras, G., Richards, R. C., Irvine, R. A., Milner, F. P. A. and Ragber, M. M. S. (1964), Infection with *Strongyloides stercoralis* in Jamaica. *Lancet*, **2**, 1257–1260.

Carr, K. E. and Toner, P. G. (1972), Surface studies of acute radiation injury in the mouse intestine. *Virchows Arch. (Zellpathol.)*, **11**, 201–210.

Cave, D. R., Mitchell, D. N. and Brooke, B. N. (1975), Observations on the transmissibility of Crohn's disease and ulcerative colitis. *Gut*, **16**, 401 (Abstract).

Cook, G. C., Kajubi, S. and Lee, F. D. (1969), Jejunal morphology of the African in Uganda. *J. Path.*, **98**, 157–169.

Dunne, W. T., Cooke, W. T. and Allan, R. N. (1977), Enzymatic and morphometric evidence for Crohn's disease as a diffuse lesion of the gastrointestinal tract. *Gut*, **18**, 290–294.

Friedman, N. B. (1945), Cellular dynamics in the intestinal mucosa: the effect of irradiation on epithelial maturation and migration. *J. exp. Med.*, **81**, 533–538.

Gangarosa, E. J., Biesil, W. R., Benyajati, C., Sprinz, H. and Pigaratu, P. (1966), The nature of the gastrointestinal lesion in Asiatic cholera and its relation to pathogenesis: a biopsy study. *Am. J. trop. Med.*, **9**, 125–135.

Greenberger, N. and Gryboski, J. D. (1973), In *Gastrointestinal Disease*, (Ed. Sleisenger, M. H. and Fordtran, J. S.), pp. 1066–1082. Saunders, Philadelphia.

Hadfield, G. (1939), The primary histological lesion of regional ileitis. *Lancet*, **2**, 773–783.

Halsted, C. H., Sheir, S. and Raasch, F. O. (1969), The small intestine in human schistosomiasis. *Gastroenterology*, **57**, 622–623.

Hawkins, C. F. (1957), Jejunal stenosis following mesenteric artery occlusion. *Lancet*, **2**, 121–122.

Knight, R., Schultz, N. G., Hoskins, D. W. and Marsden, P. D. (1973), Progress report: intestinal parasites. *Gut*, **14**, 145–168.

Kuipers, F. C., Van Theil, P. H., Rodenburg, W., Weilinga, W. J. and Roskain, R.Th. (1960), Eosinophilic phlegmon of the alimentary canal caused by a worm. *Lancet*, **2**, 1171–1173.

Lancet (1973), Intestinal capillariasis: a new disease of man. (annotation). *Lancet*, **1**, 587–588.

Lee, F. D. (1964), Pyloric metaplasia in the small intestine. *J. Path. Bact.* **87**, 267–277.

Leinbach, G. E. and Rubin, C. E. (1970), Eosinophilic gastroenteritis: a simple reaction to food allergens? *Gastroenterology*, **59**, 874–889.

Liber, A. F. (1951), Aberrant pyloric glands in regional ileitis. *Archs. Path.*, **51**, 205–212.

Mandell, H. N. (1957), Abdominal angina. Report of a case and review of the literature. *New Engl. J. Med.*, **257**, 1035–1036.

Marrash, S. E., Gibson, J. B. and Simeone, F. A. (1962), A clinico-pathologic study of intestinal infarction. *Surgery, Gynec. Obstet.*, **114**, 323–328.

Marston, A., Pheils, M. T., Thomas, M. L. and Morson, B. C. (1966), Ischaemic colitis. *Gut*, **7**, 1–5.

Meisel, J. L., Perera, D. R., Meligro, C. and Rubin, C. E. (1976), Overwhelming watery diarrhea associated with a cryptosporidium in an immunosuppressed patient. *Gastroenterology*, **70**, 1156–1160.

Morson, B. C. (1972), In *Clinics in Gastroenterology, Vol. 1, No. 3*, pp. 273–275. Saunders, London.

Nime, F. A., Burek, J. D., Page, D. L., Holscher, M. A. and Yardley, J. H. (1976), Acute enterocolitis in a human being infected with the protozoon cryptosporidium. *Gastroenterology*, **70**, 592–598.

Price, A. B. and Morson, B. C. (1975), Inflammatory bowel disease: the surgical pathology of Crohn's disease and ulcerative colitis. *Human Path.*, **6**, 7–29.

Rappaport, H., Burgoyne, F. H. and Smetana, H. F. (1951), The pathology of regional enteritis. *Milit. Surg.*, **109**, 463–502.

Reeves, R. J., Saunders, A. P., Isley, J. K., Sharpe, K. W. and Baylin, G. J. (1959), Fat absorption from the human gastrointestinal tract in patients undergoing radiation therapy. *Radiology*, **73**, 398–401.

Rickert, R. R. and Carter, H. W. (1977), The gross, light microscopic and SEM appearance of the early lesions of Crohn's disease. In *Scanning Electron Microscopy 1977/II*, 179–186. IITRI, Chicago.

Riemann, J. F. (1977), Further electron microscopic evidence of virus-like particles in Crohn's disease. *Acta Hepato-Gastroenterol.*, **24**, 116–118.

Salem, S. N. and Truelove, S. C. (1964), Hookworm disease in immigrants. *Br. med. J.*, **1**, 1074–1077.

Schreiber, D. S., Trier, J. S. and Blacklow, N. R. (1977), Recent advances in viral gastroenteritis. *Gastroenterology*, **73**, 174–183.

Sheehy, T. W., Meroney, G. H., Cox, R. S. Jnr. and Soler, J. E. (1962), Hookworm disease and malabsorption. *Gastroenterology*, **42**, 148–156.

Shiner, M. and Drury, R. A. B. (1962), Abnormalities of the small intestinal mucosa in Crohn's disease (regional enteritis). *Am. J. dig. Dis.*, **7**, 744–759.

Tankel, H. I., Clark, D. H. and Lee, F. D. (1965), Radiation enteritis with malabsorption. *Gut*, **6**, 560–569.

Trier, J. S., Moxey, R. C., Schimmel, E. M. and Robles, E. (1974), Chronic intestinal coccidiosis in man: intestinal morphology and response to treatment. *Gastroenterology*, **66**, 923–935.

Van Patter, W. N., Bargen, J. A., Dockerty, M. B., Feldman, W. H., Mayo, C. W. and Waugh, J. M. (1954), Regional enteritis. *Gastroenterology*, **26**, 347–450.

Waldmann, T. A., Wochner, R. D., Laster, L. and Gordon, R. S. (1967), Allergic gastroenteropathy. *New Engl. J. Med.*, **276**, 761–769.

Warren, S. and Sommers, S. C. (1948), Cicatrizing enteritis (regional ileitis) as a pathologic entity. *Am. J. Path.*, **24**, 475–501.

Wiernik, G. (1966), Changes in the villous pattern of the human jejunum associated with heavy radiation damage. *Gut*, **7**, 149–153.

Whalen, G. E., Rosenberg, E. B., Strickland, G. T., Gutman, R. A., Cross, J. H., Watten, R. H., Uylanogc, C. and Dizou, J. J. (1969), Intestinal capillariasis. A new disease in man. *Lancet*, **1**, 13–16.

Wright, R. G., Tomkins, A. M. and Ridley, D. S. (1977), Giardiasis: clinical and therapeutic aspects. *Gut*, **18**, 343–350.

8 Duodenitis

8.1 Evolution of the concept

The spectrum of disease processes affecting the duodenum as a whole is broadly similar to that of the remainder of the small intestine. As a result of periodic exposure to the largely unbuffered and potentially damaging effects of gastric contents, the most proximal part of the duodenum – commonly known as the duodenal bulb – provides an exception to this rule in that it may be afflicted by a series of localized pathological disturbances which more closely resemble those encountered in the stomach or distal oesophagus and are intimately, if not exclusively, related to peptic activity. The most notable of these disturbances is, of course, peptic ulceration, which is generally accepted to be the principal if not the only cause for dyspepsia of duodenal origin. The possibility that other types of pathological change in the duodenal mucosa might be responsible for dyspeptic symptoms is still regarded with suspicion by clinicians and pathologists alike.

Even so, it has been known for over 50 years that inflammatory changes are present in the mucosa surrounding peptic ulcers in the duodenum (McCarty, 1924) and that qualitatively similar changes may be found in the proximal duodenum of patients with severe dyspepsia in the absence of frank ulceration (Judd and Nagel, 1927). The long-held view that such mucosal inflammatory changes may represent a stage in the development, or regression, of duodenal ulceration (Judd and Nagel, 1927), and may be responsible for the syndrome of 'non-ulcer dyspepsia' has always, however, been difficult to establish and fell into disfavour, at least with pathologists, for many years. There were two main reasons for this. First, until quite recently the diagnosis of mucosal inflammation in the duodenum was based mainly on radiological examination, and early histological studies of random biopsies from the proximal duodenum not only showed a poor correlation with the radiological findings, but failed to provide a clear pathological basis for the syndrome of non-ulcer dyspepsia (Doniach and Shiner, 1957; Aronson and Norfleet, 1962). Secondly, it is well-recognized that duodenal ulceration may escape detection by radiological methods, and the possibility that dyspepsia might be due to an undetected ulcer could not be entirely excluded. The introduction of endoscopic techniques capable of visualizing most of the duodenal bulb have made it possible to exclude frank duodenal ulceration with greater conviction and to identify foci of mucosal congestion which may represent inflammatory change. The syndrome of non-ulcer dyspepsia has thus become more clearly defined and biopsies taken under direct visual control have provided more convincing evidence that some types of putative mucosal inflammation are related to dyspepsia and may be of relevance to the pathogenesis of peptic ulceration. The term 'duodenitis' has been widely applied to such potentially symptomatic mucosal lesions and, when employed in an unqualified fashion, implies that peptic activity is involved in its causation. Perhaps the term 'peptic duodenitis' would be more appropriate to avoid confusion with other known causes of duodenal inflammation such as infective gastro-enteritis or Crohn's disease.

The histological definition of 'duodenitis' nevertheless presents considerable difficulties, not least as a result of the considerable variation in villous pattern and leucocytic infiltration observed in the mucosa of the duodenal bulb in apparently normal individuals, and there is little general agreement as to which histological features are significant either pathologically or with regard to clinical symptoms. Perhaps the best that can be done at the moment is to analyse the features which, at one time or another, have been considered important.

8.2 Histological changes attributed to duodenitis

8.2.1 Oedema and congestion

Although these are classical signs of inflammation, their presence is not of much diagnostic value to the histopathologist since operative artefact can never be entirely excluded. They are, however, of greater use to the endoscopist in identifying foci of mucosal inflammation, and it has been reported that there is quite a good correlation between 'macroscopic' mucosal congestion and histological evidence of 'inflammation' (Cotton et al., 1973).

8.2.2 Increased 'round-cell' infiltration

Increased 'round-cell' infiltration in the lamina propria – by which is meant an increase in plasma cells, eosinophils and lymphocytes (see the 'non-specific response' Section 4.1.3) – is mentioned in most studies on duodenitis, and has been used as a method for grading the severity of inflammatory change and assessing the response of the mucosa to treatment designed to lower acid output (Beck *et al.*, 1965; Rhodes *et al.*, 1968). The validity of this change as a sole indication of duodenitis is however open to question, since in any individual case it is difficult to decide the exact point at which mucosal leucocytic infiltration becomes abnormal. Increased round cell infiltration in the mucosa was judged to be present in 25 per cent of normal control biopsies in one series (Cotton *et al.*, 1973) and only in unusually severe cases can it be regarded as unequivocally pathological (Fig. 8.1). Moreover, this type of change is entirely non-specific and may be an expression of a more diffuse reaction in the intestinal mucosa as takes place, for example, in coeliac disease.

8.2.3 *Neutrophil infiltration*

The emigration of neutrophils into the lamina propria, epithelial surface or crypt lumina of the duodenal mucosa is thought to be a more reliable marker for the presence of an inflammatory process as there is no evidence that these changes can be attributed to traumatic artefact (Cotton *et al.*, 1973), which at most only produces margination of polymorphs within blood vessels. Neutrophil emigration implies that some degree of epithelial damage is taking place (Section 4.1.3) and, when there is morphological evidence of this, the term 'active duodenitis' has been applied (Cotton *et al.*, 1973). While this change is not necessarily a consequence of peptic activity, it is not often prominent in other forms of intestinal inflammatory disease likely to involve the duodenum (see Section 4.1.3). On the other hand, 'active duodenitis' is commonly seen in the vicinity of chronic peptic ulcers in the duodenum.

8.2.4 *Epithelial changes*

The epithelial damage referred to in association with 'active duodenitis' is revealed by the presence of cytoplasmic basophilia, nuclear hyperchromatism and irregularity, reduction in cell height and sometimes 'tufting' or syncytial change (Fig. 4.10). Foci of superficial erosion may also be observed (Fig. 8.3). It is most improbable that traumatic artefact could reproduce such changes, which have been regarded as undoubtedly pathological in any circumstances. They are not, however, specific for duodenitis: almost identical changes may be

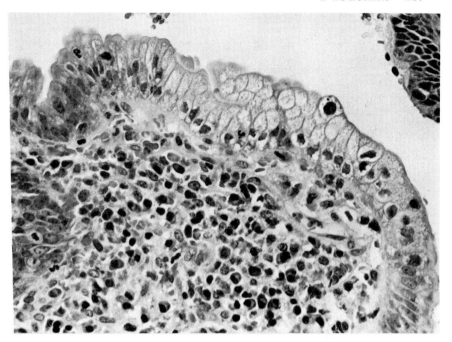

Fig. 8.1 Active duodenitis. In this endoscopic duodenal biopsy the surface epithelium shows cytoplasmic vacuolation and nuclear irregularity, and occasional neutrophils are seen within the epithelial surface. There is also a marked increase in leucocytes in the lamina propria. HE × 450.

found in coeliac disease and in other diseases which produce the atrophic villous pattern (Section 4.2.1).

8.2.5 Changes in villous architecture

In the normal duodenal bulb, the villi tend to be shorter and more leaf-shaped, and the crypts more elongated than elsewhere in the small intestine (Fig. 8.2). This would suggest that the enterocyte lifespan is marginally reduced when compared with the jejunum, possibly as a result of the more variable chemical environment. Considerable variability of villous pattern is also observed in apparently normal individuals, and even within the same biopsy specimen (cf. Figs. 8.2 and 8.4). As a result of this, only a severe degree of villous atrophy of crypt hyperplastic type can be regarded as unequivocally abnormal in the proximal duodenum. Random biopsy studies of the duodenal bulb have shown that while significant villous atrophy is common in association with frank duodenal ulceration, it is much less conspicuous

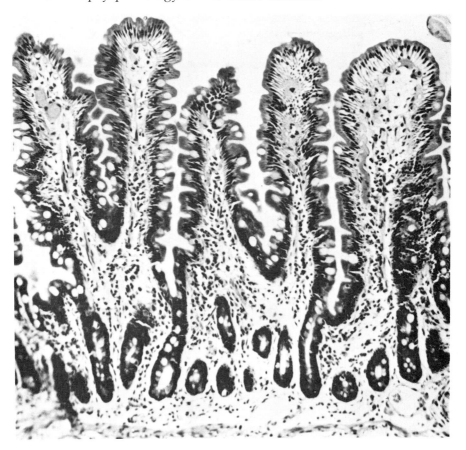

Fig. 8.2 Normal duodenum. The villi tend to be shorter and the crypts more elongated than in the normal jejunum (cf. Fig. 8.4). HE × 180.

in cases of non-ulcer dyspepsia (Gear and Dobbins, 1969); and in endoscopic studies of supposed foci of duodenitis villous atrophy is a most variable feature and is pronounced only in a minority of cases (Fig. 8.3). As might be expected villous atrophy, when present, is usually associated with evidence of epithelial damage, although there is not always a close correlation between these two changes. Moreover, villous atrophy, even in the proximal duodenum, is not a specific expression of peptic activity; there is a real possibility that coeliac disease and other causes of the atrophic villous pattern (Section 4.2.1) may produce similar changes in this area.

8.2.6 Metaplastic change

In the duodenal bulb, metaplastic change can only be readily recognized by the replacement of enterocytes at the villous extremity by groups of epithelial cells with the morphological and staining characteristics of gastric surface epithelium (James, 1964; Fig. 4.10). This is usually associated with the incursion of Brunners glands into the mucosa (Fig. 8.4) and there can be little doubt that the metaplastic changes originate in the crypts, as is the case elsewhere in the small bowel (Section 4.1.2). Metaplasia is present in the duodenal bulb in well over half of cases of duodenal ulceration (James, 1964) and there is experimental evidence to suggest that it is a manifestation of hyperchlorhydria (Rhodes, 1964). It has also been reported in about one third of patients with non-ulcer dyspepsia (Cotton *et al.*, 1973) and it is interesting that Brunner gland hyperplasia has also been described in this condition (Stokes *et al.*, 1964). Metaplasia is commonly associated with some degree of villous atrophy (Gear and Dobbins, 1969), but it correlates less well with evidence of active inflammation; this would

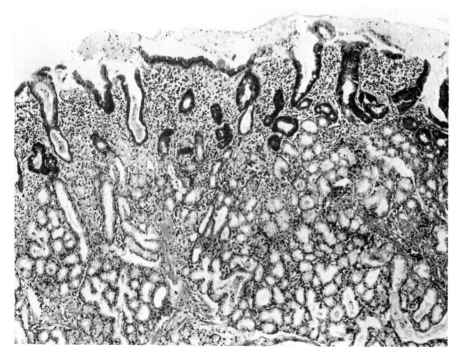

Fig. 8.3 Active duodenitis. There is villous blunting. Increased leucocytic infiltration in the lamina propria and foci of superficial mucosal erosion are seen. HE × 70.

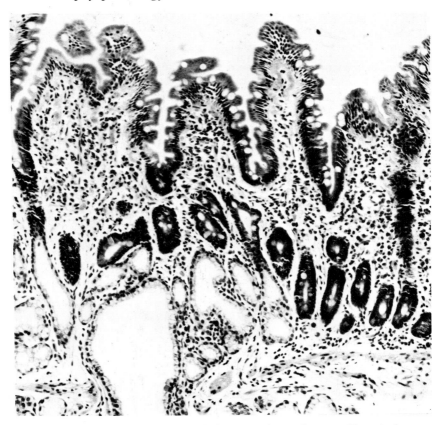

Fig. 8.4 Normal duodenum. The villi are irregular in shape and length due to extension of Brunners glands into the mucosa. This is the same biopsy as illustrated in Fig. 8.2. HE × 180.

support the possibility that metaplastic change is fundamentally a protective device.

8.3 Comment

It is apparent from this assessment that there is still uncertainty with regard to the histopathological definition of duodenitis, and that the pathogenesis of non-ulcer dyspepsia has yet to be fully elucidated. This uncertainty is most readily illustrated by the difficulties encountered in interpreting the most obvious sign of mucosal inflammation, namely, an increase in round-cell infiltration of the lamina propria. While this change may be statistically significant when groups of patients with dyspepsia are compared with normal individuals (Beck *et al.*, 1965), it is much too variable and non-specific a factor to be of diagnostic value in individual cases. Moreover, as in the case of chronic gastritis, it has yet to be shown that it is capable of producing dyspeptic symptoms. Precisely the same comments may be applied to villous atrophy. Although it is possible that foci of severe villous atrophy may indicate sites of incipient or healing ulceration in the duodenum, it has always been notoriously difficult to assess the meaning of changes in villous architecture in the proximal duodenum.

The lesion referred to as 'active duodenitis' is characterized by the migration of neutrophil polymorphs into the mucosal lamina propria or across epithelial surfaces. This abnormality, often accompanied by evidence of damage to the enterocyte population, has a greater claim to being unequivocally pathological. It also seems to correlate better than other changes with the presence of dyspeptic symptoms (Cotton *et al.*, 1973). It is not without relevance that the symptoms of gastro-oesophageal reflux similarly correlate better with signs of epithelial embarrassment than with leucocyte alterations in the lamina propria of the distal oesophagus (Ismail-Beigi *et al.*, 1970). It must be emphasized, however, that the clinical implications of 'active duodenitis' have yet to be fully evaluated, and its diagnostic specificity remains uncertain; it is possible that factors other than peptic activity may be involved in its causation.

The position with regard to gastric metaplasia in the duodenal bulb is somewhat different. While there is convincing evidence that this change is related to high acid levels in the duodenum, it is not necessarily associated with signs of mucosal inflammation, nor can it be regarded per se as a cause of dyspeptic symptoms. On the other hand, when metaplasia is associated with inflammatory change and especially with active duodenitis, it provides presumptive evidence that peptic activity is responsible for the inflammatory change. The presence of metaplasia may also be helpful in identifying patients with a high risk of developing peptic ulceration in the duodenum. In this context, it is notable that active duodenitis, and other histological changes associated with duodenitis such as gastric metaplasia and villous atrophy, are also found in patients with peptic ulceration. They indeed tend to be more conspicuous. Thus the long-held view that duodenal ulceration might be preceded by peptic duodenitis retains validity, and recent follow-up studies of patients with symptomatic active duodenitis tend to support this concept (Thomson *et al.*, 1977).

8.4 Summary

While it is tempting to conclude that 'active' duodenitis forms the basis of the syndrome of non-ulcer dyspepsia and that it represents a phase in the evolution of peptic ulceration in the duodenum, further controlled biopsy studies are clearly necessary. Direct comparison between inflamed and non-inflamed mucosa identified by endoscopy of the duodenal bulb may help to overcome the problems of histological variation between individuals and to establish more clearly the clinical significance not only of 'active' duodenitis but also of more 'chronic' forms of duodenitis characterized by increased round-cell infiltration in the lamina propria. Such 'auto-control' studies may also be helpful in distinguishing between 'peptic' forms of duodenitis, which appear to be focal or patchy in distribution, and more diffuse forms of mucosal inflammation as typified by coeliac disease.

References

Aronson, A. R. and Norfleet, R. G. (1962), The duodenal mucosal in peptic ulcer disease: a clinical pathological correlation. *Am. J. dig. Dis.*, **7**, 506–514.

Beck, I. T., Kahn, D. S., Lacerte, M., Solymar, J., Callegarini, V. and Geokas, M. C. with the assistance of Phelps, E. (1965), Chronic duodenitis: a clinical pathological entity? *Gut*, **6**, 376–383.

Cotton, P. B., Price, A. B., Tighe, J. R. and Beales, J. S. M. (1973), Preliminary evaluation of 'duodenitis' by endoscopy and biopsy. *Br. med. J.*, **3**, 430–433.

Doniach, I. and Shiner, M. (1957), Duodenal and jejunal biopsies. II. Histology. *Gastroenterology*, **33**, 71–86.

Gear, E. V. and Dobbins, W. O. (1969), The histological spectrum of proximal duodenal biopsy in adult males. *Am. J. med. Sci.*, **257**, 90–99.

Ismail-Beigi, F., Horton, P. F. and Pope, C. E. II (1970), Histological consequences of gastro-esophageal reflux in man. *Gastroenterology*, **58**, 163–174.

James, A. H. (1964), Gastric epithelium in the duodenum. *Gut*, **5**, 285–294.

Judd, E. D. and Nagel, G. W. (1927), Excision of ulcer of duodenum. *Surgery, Gynec. Obstet.*, **45**, 17–23.

McCarty, W. C. (1924), Excised duodenal ulcers: a report of four hundred and twenty-five specimens. *J. Am. med. Ass.*, **83**, 1894–1898.

Rhodes, J. (1964), Experimental production of gastric epithelium in the duodenum. *Gut*, **5**, 454–458.

Rhodes, J., Evans, K. T., Lawrie, J. H. and Forrest, A. P. M. (1968), Coarse mucosal folds in the duodenum. *Q. J. Med.*, **37**, 151–169.

Stokes, J. F., Turnberg, L. A. and Hawksley, J. C. (1964), Hyperplasia of Brunner's glands. *Gut*, **5**, 459–462.

Thomson, W. O., Robertson, A. G., Imrie, C. W., Joffe, S. N., Lee, F. D. and Blumgart, L. H. (1977), Is duodenitis a dyspeptic myth? *Lancet*, **1**, 1197–1198.

9 Tumours of the small intestine

Neoplastic processes are much less often a cause of clinical disturbance in the small bowel than in the other parts of the gastro-intestinal tract, and with certain exceptions random intestinal biopsy is seldom of value in diagnosis. A detailed description of neoplasms of the small bowel would thus be inappropriate in a discussion of biopsy pathology. Nevertheless most types of intestinal neoplasia may affect the upper duodenum and may on occasion become accessible to endoscopic visualization and biopsy. A brief account of the more important intestinal tumours follows.

9.1 Connective tissue tumours

While it is difficult to assess the true incidence of these tumours, only rarely can clinical symptoms be attributed to them. The smooth muscle tumours, leiomyoma and leiomyosarcoma are perhaps the least rare and are well-organized, if uncommon, cause of cryptic intestinal blood loss. Sometimes like other polypoid tumours, both epithelial and mesenchymal, they produce intussusception. Malignancy can only be proved when metastasis can be demonstrated, but when mitotic activity can be found in every high power microscopic field the tumour should be regarded as having malignant potential. Lymphangioma (Fig. 9.1) is a harmless lesion which is usually discovered accidentally in the proximal small bowel during gastric operations or endoscopy. Haemangiomas, less common and occasionally multiple, may be a cause of intestinal blood loss; of more importance in this respect, however, are the mucosal vascular malformations found in hereditary haemorrhagic telangiectasia. Rarely, neural tumours, both benign and malignant, may be found as part of generalized neurofibromatosis, and mucosal neuromas may also be found in one variant of the multiple endocrine adenoma syndrome (MEA2 or Sipple syndrome).

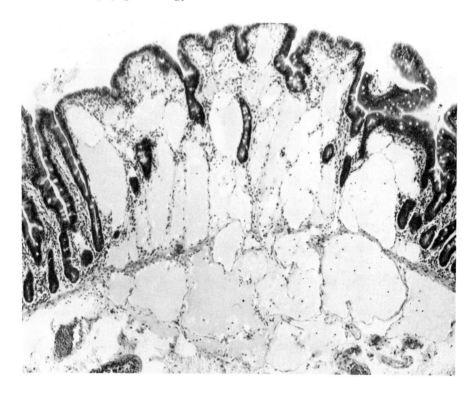

Fig. 9.1 Lymphangioma of duodenum. There is focal aggregation of cavernous lymphatic channels producing localized villous distortion. HE × 90.

9.2 Epithelial tumours

The rarity of epithelial tumours in the small bowel is still unexplained. Benign tumours comparable to the 'neoplastic polypi' of adenomatous or papillary type in the colon are particularly uncommon, although simple adenomas have on occasion been diagnosed in biopsies carried out during endoscopic visualization of the duodenum (Fig. 9.2). The tumour illustrated arose close to the ampulla of Vater and produced obstructive jaundice (Fig. 9.3). The intestinal polypi which characterize

Fig. 9.2 Simple adenoma of duodenum. There is hyperchromatism and loss of polarity of the neoplastic epithelial cells. Paneth cell differentiation is also a prominent feature. HE × 450.
Fig. 9.3 Simple adenoma of duodenum. A low-power view of a tumour which produced obstruction of the common bile duct at the ampulla of Vater. HE × 45.

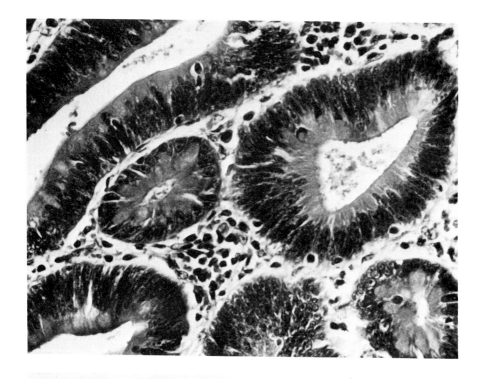

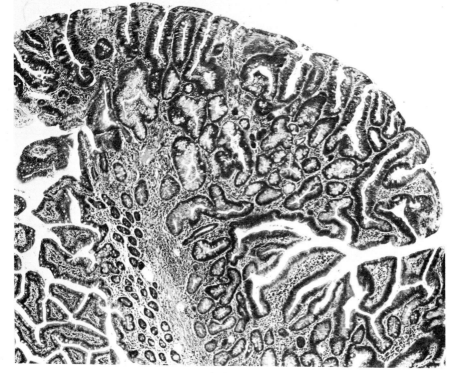

the Peutz-Jeghers syndrome are now generally regarded as hamartomatous rather than neoplastic in nature. The 'juvenile' polypi which
occasionally involve the small intestine may also be hamartomatous.
Adenocarcinoma of the small intestine (which length for length is most
common in the duodenum) has much the same general features as the
more common colonic forms of carcinoma, and presents a similar
histological appearance. The peculiar type of carcinoma which may
complicate Crohn's disease of the small bowel deserves special mention (Fleming and Pollock, 1975). The 'endometrioid' infiltrative
pattern, with apparently isolated acinar structures penetrating the
thickened bowel wall, is distinctive; but of greater relevance to
biopsy pathology is the presence of severe dysplasia of the overlying villous epithelium, a feature of potential diagnostic importance
(Fig. 9.4).

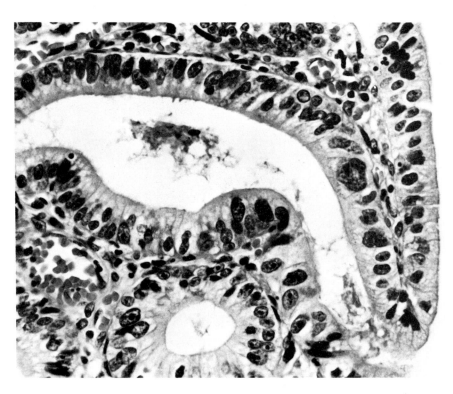

Fig. 9.4 Crohn's disease. In this case, an ileal resection showed that the disease
was complicated by an infiltrative carcinoma, and the epithelium on the
mucosal surface showed marked dysplastic change. HE × 510.

9.3 Malignant lymphoid tumours

These tumours are of particular importance in the small intestine, where they are at least as common as primary carcinomas. The intestine may, of course, be involved secondarily during the course of a systematized lymphoma (Cornes et al., 1961) or in leukaemic states, including the Sézary syndrome (Cohen et al., 1977), but, in most instances, intestinal lymphomas arise primarily in the gut-associated lymphoid tissues. The tendency of these primary lymphomas to produce intestinal perforation is well-recognized (Irvine and Johnstone, 1955) and another feature requiring emphasis is the frequency with which multiple lesions develop. Sometimes more than one intestinal tumour is found at the time of clinical presentation; in other instances recurrence of tumour may take place some considerable time after initial surgical resection, as long as 5 years in one personally observed case. Whether these phenomena result from metastasis or from multifocal tumour formation is uncertain. While intestinal lymphomas may spread to the mesenteric lymph nodes, and sometimes to more distant sites such as liver, spleen and bone marrow, the prognosis is not always hopeless since in a substantial proportion of cases there is no evidence of metastasis at the time of surgical resection.

The aetiology of primary intestinal lymphomas is unknown. Nevertheless it is now well-established that there is a relationship between this tumour and malabsorptive states, especially coeliac disease, as first suggested by Gough et al. (1962). The evidence for this comes from two main sources. First, long-term follow-up studies of patients proven by clinical and pathological methods to have coeliac disease have shown a significant increase in the incidence of intestinal lymphoma, as well as other tumours such as oesophageal carcinoma (Harris et al., 1967). Secondly, diffuse villous atrophy of the intestinal mucosa is commonly observed in association with lymphomas in surgical resections, even when there is no clear history of malabsorption prior to surgery (Lee, 1966; Brunt et al., 1969). The significance of these mucosal changes has been discussed in an earlier section (Section 5.1) but it seems probable that in most cases they are due to unrecognized coeliac disease. If this is correct, the results of pathological studies of intestinal lymphomas reviewed personally in the West of Scotland would suggest that about 40 per cent of these tumours are related to coeliac disease, and this percentage is substantially greater if only lymphomas of the proximal small bowel are considered.

Certain pathological features of coeliac disease appear to be especially associated with the development of lymphoma, and these may be particularly relevant to biopsy assessment. Of special interest in this respect is the complication of non-specific ulceration ('ulcerative jejunitis'), which is becoming increasingly recognized as a pre-lymphomatous condition (Whitehead, 1968; Isaacson and Wright, 1978). Pronounced subepithelial collagen deposition ('collagenous sprue') may also be associated with both ulceration and lymphoma (Jeffries *et al.*, 1968; Whitehead, 1971). The presence in a random jejunal biopsy of an unusually dense leucocytic infiltrate in the lamina propria, especially when accompanied by an increase in small lympho-cytes or atypical 'reticulum cells' ('progressive hyperplasia'; see Whitehead, 1971), may also raise the suspicion that lymphoma may develop (Ferguson *et al.*, 1974). In some personally studied cases of lymphoma there has also been a massive increase in intra-epithelial lymphocytes in the related mucosa (Figs. 5.13 and 5.14).

In general, lymphoma appears to arise more often in the distal, as opposed to the proximal, small bowel (see Read, 1970). The distribu-tion of the various histological types of lymphoma involved is still a controversial matter. Early studies suggested that 'large lymphoid' tumours ('reticulosarcoma') accounted for just over half of all intestinal lymphomas and 'small lymphoid' tumours ('lymphosarcoma') for about one third, the remainder, including Hodgkin's disease, being uncommon (Read, 1970). More recent studies, however, have pre-sented evidence that primary Hodgkin's disease of the small bowel is extremely rare, and that nearly half of all lymphomas are of plasma-cell type, 'large lymphoid' tumours, lymphocytic, lymphoblastic and ger-minal centre tumours accounting for most of the remainder (Henry and Farrer-Brown, 1977). The tumours associated with coeliac disease, or with diffuse villous atrophy, present a somewhat different picture. Almost all such tumours arise in the upper small bowel (see Read, 1970; Austad *et al.*, 1967; Harris *et al.*, 1967) and the great majority are of 'large lymphoid' type (reticulosarcoma). Indeed, it has been suggested recently that almost all of these tumours are of histiocytic origin, and the possibility raised that the ulceration which quite often precedes lymphoma is caused by 'self-destructing' multifocal histiocytic growths (Isaacson and Wright, 1978). It may also be speculated that the unusual forms of mucosal lymphocytic infiltration observed to precede lym-phoma (see above) may represent an attempt to combat the establish-ment of histiocytic lymphoma. A notable feature of 'coeliac lym-phomas' is the frequency with which the tumour cells are accompanied by a pleomorphic infiltrate of lymphocytes, plasma cells and eosinophils. This phenomenon may well account for the probably erroneous suggestion that Hodgkin's disease of the small bowel or mesenteric nodes may complicate coeliac disease (Read, 1970; Austad *et al.*, 1967).

Malabsorption may result from a different mechanism in the so-called 'Mediterranean' type of intestinal lymphoma which has been described in many parts of the Middle East and may be found in immigrants in Britain (Doe *et al.*, 1972). While the types of lymphoma usually encountered in Europe or North America are distinctly focal (or multifocal) tumours, the Mediterranean type characteristically involves the intestinal mucosa in a diffuse fashion, often affecting the entire length of the small bowel. Malabsorption is thus a direct consequence of tumour growth, which can usually be detected by dense infiltration of the lamina propria by tumour cells, most of which resemble plasma cells or plasmacytoid lymphocytes (Fig. 9.5). While the appearances resemble coeliac disease, the sparsity of the crypts and the presence in advanced cases of nucleolated blast cells in the leucocytic infiltrate enable the distinction to be made. A further phenome-

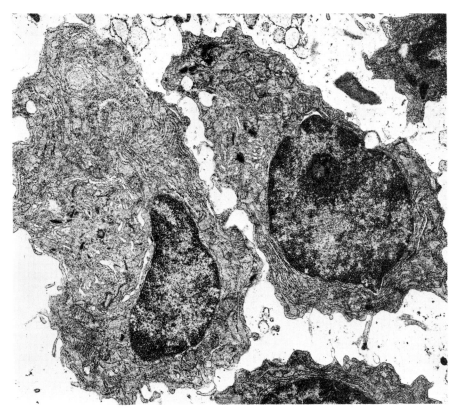

Fig. 9.5 Plasmacytoid cells from a case of α-chain disease. These cells have the elaborate granular endoplasmic reticulum and Golgi systems of typical plasma cells. Micrograph by courtesy of Dr A. Galian. (Galian *et al.*, 1977.)

non of diagnostic value is the presence in some cases of the heavy alpha chain of IgA immunoglobulin in the serum (α-chain disease; Rambaud et al., 1968; Galian et al., 1977).

Systemic mast cell disease may also be detected on rare occasions by intestinal biopsy. Malabsorption may be a feature of this condition, although its cause is uncertain. In some cases at least, malabsorption has been due to co-existent coeliac disease. (Scott et al., 1975.)

9.4 Tumours of the intestinal endocrine system

This system consists of a series of endocrine cells which, although residing within the epithelial surface of the gastro-intestinal tract, are thought by some to be of neural crest origin. A currently popular name for these cells, the APUD system, derives from a property common to the constituent cell types, namely amine precursor uptake and decarboxylation. The cells also produce polypeptide hormones (see Section 3.3). At least eight different types of gastro-intestinal endocrine cells have been described (Pearse, 1977; Pearse et al., 1977): the tumours of this endocrine system vary in their secretory capacity and in the histochemical properties of the constituent cells. The most common type is the classical 'carcinoid' tumour which is derived from the EC (enterochromaffin) cell. The tumour cells usually exhibit the characteristic histological argentaffin reaction. In the small intestine these tumours may be multiple and tend to behave as low-grade carcinomas, invading the mesentery and metastasizing to the mesenteric lymph nodes and liver. Systemic effects attributable to the formation of amines and other secretory products by the tumour cells (the carcinoid syndrome) only develop when there is extensive metastasis to the liver. Diarrhoea and more rarely malabsorption may be features of the classical carcinoid syndrome, and may also be found in association with other intestinal endocrine tumours such as pancreatic vasoactive intestinal peptide (VIP) secreting tumours (vipomas; Bloom, Polak and Pearse, 1973). Intestinal biopsy, however, is usually without diagnostic value in such cases, so that further consideration of the subject would be inappropriate in this book.

References

Austad, W. I., Cornes, J. S., Gough, K. R., McCarthy, C. F. and Read, A. E. (1967), Steatorrhoea and malignant lymphoma. The relationship of malignant tumours of lymphoid tissue and coeliac disease. Am. J. dig. Dis., 12, 475–490.

Bloom, S. R., Polak, J. M. and Pearse, A. G. E. (1973), Vasoactive intestinal peptide and watery-diarrhoea syndrome. *Lancet*, **2**, 14–16.

Brunt, P. W., Sircus, W. and McLean, N. (1969), Neoplasia and the coeliac syndrome in adults. *Lancet*, **I**, 180–184.

Cohen, M. I., Wilderlite, L. W., Schechter, G. P., Jaffe, E., Fischmann, A. B., Schein, P. S. and MacDonald, J. S. (1977), Gastrointestinal involvement in the Sézary syndrome. *Gastroenterology*, **73**, 145–149.

Cornes, J. S., Jones, T. G. and Fisher, G. B. (1961), Gastroduodenal ulceration and massive haemorrhage in patients with leukaemia, multiple myeloma and malignant tumours of lymphoid tissue. *Gastroenterology*, **41**, 337–344.

Doe, W. F., Henry, K., Hobbs, J. R., Avery Jones, F., Dent, C. E. and Booth, C. C. (1972), Five cases of alpha-chain disease. *Gut*, **13**, 947–957.

Ferguson, R., Asquith, P. and Cooke, W. T. (1974), The jejunal cellular infiltrate in coeliac disease complicated by lymphoma. *Gut*, **15**, 458–461.

Fleming, K. A. and Pollock, A. C. (1975), A case of 'Crohn's carcinoma'. *Gut*, **16**, 533–537.

Galian, A., Lecestre, M. J., Scotto, J., Bognel, C., Matuchancky, C. and Rambaud, J-C. (1977), Pathological study of alpha-chain disease, with special emphasis on evolution. *Cancer*, **39**, 2081–2101.

Gough, K. R., Read, A. E. and Naish, J. M. (1962), Intestinal reticulosis as a complication of idiopathic steatorrhoea. *Gut*, **3**, 232–239.

Harris, O. D., Cooke, W. T., Thompson, H. and Waterhouse, J. A. H. (1967), Malignancy in adult coeliac disease and idiopathic steatorrhoea. *Am. J. Med.*, **42**, 899–912.

Henry, K. and Farrer-Brown, G. (1977), Primary lymphomas of the gastrointestinal tract. I. Plasma cell tumours. *Histopathology*, **1**, 53–76.

Irvine, W. T. and Johnstone, J. M. (1955), Lymphosarcoma of the small intestine: with special reference to perforating tumours. *Br. J. Surg.*, **42**, 611–617.

Isaacson, P. and Wright, D. H. (1978), Intestinal lymphoma associated with malabsorption. *Lancet*, **1**, 67–70.

Jeffries, G. H., Steinberg, H. and Sleisenger, M. H. (1968), Chronic ulcerative (non-granulomatous) jejunitis. *Am. J. Med.*, **44**, 47–59.

Lee, F. D. (1966), The nature of the mucosal changes associated with malignant tumours of the small intestine. *Gut*, **7**, 361–367.

Pearse, A. G. E. (1977), In *The Gastrointestinal Tract*, (Ed. Yardley, J. H., Morson, B. C. and Abell, M. R.) The Williams and Wilkins Co., Baltimore.

Pearse, A. G. E., Polak, J. M. and Bloom, S. R. (1977), The newer gut hormones. Cellular sources, physiology, pathology and clinical aspects. *Gastroenterology*, **72**, 746–761.

Rambaud, J. C., Bognel, C., Prost, A., Burnier, J. L. Le Quintrec, Y., Lambling, A., Danon, F., Hurez, D. and Seligmann, M. (1968), Clinico-pathological study of a patient with 'Mediterranean' type of abdominal lymphoma and a new type of IgA abnormality ('Alpha Chain Disease'). *Digestion*, **1**, 321–336.

Read, A. E. (1970), In *Modern Trends in Gastroenterology* No. 4, (Ed. Card, W. I. and Creamer, B.). Butterworths, London.

Scott, B. B., Hardy, G. J. and Losowsky, M. S. (1975), Involvement of the small intestine in systemic mast cell disease. *Gut*, **16**, 918–924.

Whitehead, R. (1968), Primary lymphadenopathy complicating idiopathic steatorrhea. *Gut*, **9**, 569–575.

Whitehead, R. (1971), The interpretation and significance of morphological abnormalities in jejunal biopsies. In *Intestinal Absorption and its Derangements*. (Ed. Dawson, A. M.) *J. clin. Path.*, **24**, Suppl. (Roy. Coll. Path.), **5**, 108–124.

Index

Figures in *italics* refer to pages with illustrations: **bold** figures indicate the major entry for the topic.